AF788187

Pharmacovigilance - Facts, Challenges, Limitations and Opportunities

Edited by Farid A. Badria

Published in London, United Kingdom

Pharmacovigilance - Facts, Challenges, Limitations and Opportunities
http://dx.doi.org/10.5772/intechopen.1003318
Edited by Farid A. Badria

Contributors
Abdullah A. Elgazar, Aivle Libertad Hernández Caamaño, Anant Khot, Dhanya Sacheendran, Fan Li, Farid A. Badria, Ganesh Dakhale, Ivo Abraham, Jian Yang, Karla Roman Flores, Mamatha Jayachandran, Martin Kondža, Miguel Luján Estrada, Mohamed Gamaleldin, Princy Louis Palatty, Shaimaa Abdelhalim

© The Editor(s) and the Author(s) 2025
The rights of the editor(s) and the author(s) have been asserted in accordance with the Copyright, Designs and Patents Act 1988. All rights to the book as a whole are reserved by INTECHOPEN LIMITED. The book as a whole (compilation) cannot be reproduced, distributed or used for commercial or non-commercial purposes without INTECHOPEN LIMITED's written permission. Enquiries concerning the use of the book should be directed to INTECHOPEN LIMITED rights and permissions department (permissions@intechopen.com).
Violations are liable to prosecution under the governing Copyright Law.

CC BY

Individual chapters of this publication are distributed under the terms of the Creative Commons Attribution 4.0 License which permits commercial use, distribution and reproduction of the individual chapters, provided the original author(s) and source publication are appropriately acknowledged. If so indicated, certain images may not be included under the Creative Commons license. In such cases users will need to obtain permission from the license holder to reproduce the material. More details and guidelines concerning content reuse and adaptation can be found at http://www.intechopen.com/ copyright-policy.html.

Notice
Statements and opinions expressed in the chapters are these of the individual contributors and not necessarily those of the editors or publisher. No responsibility is accepted for the accuracy of information contained in the published chapters. The publisher assumes no responsibility for any damage or injury to persons or property arising out of the use of any materials, instructions, methods or ideas contained in the book.

First published in London, United Kingdom, 2025 by IntechOpen
IntechOpen is the global imprint of INTECHOPEN LIMITED, registered in England and Wales, registration number: 11086078, 167-169 Great Portland Street, London, W1W 5PF, United Kingdom

For EU product safety concerns: IN TECH d.o.o., Prolaz Marije Krucifikse Kozulić 3, 51000 Rijeka, Croatia, info@intechopen.com or visit our website at intechopen.com.

British Library Cataloguing-in-Publication Data
A catalogue record for this book is available from the British Library

Pharmacovigilance - Facts, Challenges, Limitations and Opportunities
Edited by Farid A. Badria
p. cm.

This title is part of the Pharmaceutical Science Book Series, Volume 11
Topic: Pharmacology
Series Editor: Rosario Pignatello
Topic Editor: Cristina Manuela Drăgoi
Associate Topic Editor: Alina Crenguţa Nicolae

Print ISBN 978-0-85466-563-1
Online ISBN 978-0-85466-562-4
eBook (PDF) ISBN 978-0-85466-564-8
ISSN 3033-3318

If disposing of this product, please recycle the paper responsibly.

We are IntechOpen, the world's leading publisher of Open Access books

Built by scientists, for scientists

7,500+
Open access books available

195,000+
International authors and editors

215M+
Downloads

156
Countries delivered to

Our authors are among the
Top 1%
most cited scientists

12.2%
Contributors from top 500 universities

CLARIVATE ANALYTICS BOOK CITATION INDEX INDEXED

WEB OF SCIENCE™

Selection of our books indexed in the Book Citation Index in Web of Science™ Core Collection (BKCI)

Interested in publishing with us? Contact book.department@intechopen.com

Numbers displayed above are based on latest data collected.
For more information visit www.intechopen.com

IntechOpen Book Series
Pharmaceutical Science
Volume 11

Aims and Scope of the Series

Pharmaceutical science focuses on the design, synthesis, formulation, targeting, distribution, safety, and efficacy of active compounds as potential therapeutics. It is a large interdisciplinary discipline that aims to integrate the basic principles of physical and organic chemistry, biochemistry, biology, and engineering to discover, develop, and characterize active compounds and to optimize the formulation and delivery of drugs in the body for offering new and improved safe and efficacious therapies against human diseases. The research areas covered by the pharmaceutical sciences range from medicinal chemistry and pharmaceutical technology to pharmacology and toxicology, which represent the preliminary phases of drug development. Medicinal chemistry involves the design and synthesis of pharmaceuticals as well as the isolation of active agents from natural sources. Computer-aided strategies are increasingly involved in this drug discovery process. Pharmaceutics is a multidisciplinary science that examines the relationships between drug formulation, delivery, distribution, and clinical outcomes. Modern clinical approaches are increasingly relying on controlled release strategies and drug delivery and targeting systems, including nanotechnological platforms (nanomedicine). Pharmacology is the science of drug action in biological systems. Pharmacologists also make drugs as tools to explore aspects of cell and tissue functions. Toxicology is the study of the adverse effects of active agents on living organisms and the ecosystem, including the prevention and amelioration of such adverse effects. This book series includes volumes on Drug Discovery, Delivery, and Pharmacology. Their overall aim is to present the latest research in the whole path of drug discovery and development from different points of view of this multidisciplinary and dynamic field.

Meet the Series Editor

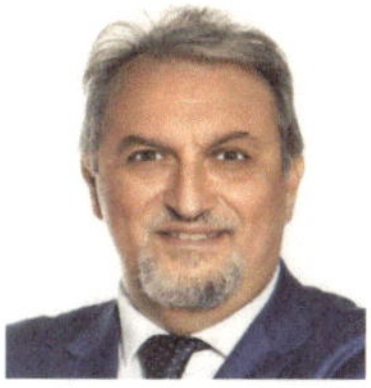

Prof. Rosario Pignatello is a Full Professor of Pharmaceutical Technology and Legislation at the University of Catania, Italy. He is the Director of the Department of Drug and Health Sciences. He has nearly 30 years of experience in the research and development of innovative formulations for the controlled release and targeting of bioactive molecules, through chemical approaches as well as nanotechnological carriers, aimed at treating different disorders. Prof. Pignatello has coauthored about 180 papers and edited a series of textbooks on biomaterials and their application in medicine. The main areas of his research are polymeric and lipid-based micro- and nanoparticles as modified drug delivery systems; vesicular nanocarriers (liposomes, micelles); lipophilic prodrugs and conjugates; synthesis and evaluation of new polymeric biomaterials for drug delivery and tissue regeneration. In particular, Prof. Pignatello works actively in the field of ocular drug delivery, leading the Research Centre for Ocular Nanotechnology, within the NANOMED Centre (Centre for Nanomedicine and Pharmaceutical Nanotechnology) at the University of Catania.

Meet the Volume Editor

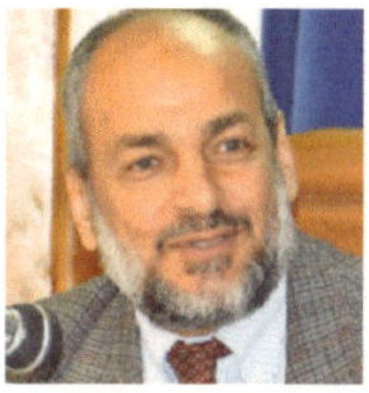

Professor Farid Badria, Ph.D., DSc, leads research projects on developing new liver, skin disorders, and cancer therapies. According to the lists published by Stanford University, USA, he was among the top 2% of the most-cited scientists in medicinal and biomolecular chemistry in 2019-2022. He has been a scholar with the Arab Development Fund, Kuwait, ICRO-UNESCO, Chile, and UNESCO Biotechnology, France. He has received the TWAS Prize for the Public Understanding of Science, the WIPO Gold Medal for the best inventor, the State Outstanding Award in Medicine, the Outstanding Arab Scholar, Kuwait, and the Khawrazmi International Award, Iran. Prof. Badria has over 270 publications, including twelve books, has submitted 49 patents, 20 of which have received final certification, and has marketed several pharmaceutical products.

Contents

Preface

Medication safety, often known as pharmacovigilance (from the words pharmakon and vigilare), is a science that deals with the "collection, detection, assessment, monitoring, and prevention" of adverse medication effects. Even after a medication or treatment has been available for a while, it is always crucial to keep an eye out for side effects because new ones could appear. It is important to remember that an unpleasant reaction is distinguished from an adverse event by the suspicion of a direct association between a medical product and an incident. Additionally, pharmacovigilance has three stages: pre-clinical, clinical trial, and post-marketing. Every stage has an impact on guaranteeing the security of medications. Alternatively, the pharmacovigilance process could include the following steps: stage 1: Detection. Gathering Individual Case Safety Reports (ICSRs), Phase 2: Evaluation, Phase 3: Comprehending the pharmacological safety profile, and Phase 4: Avoiding negative consequences.

This book aims to provide pharmaceutical companies with good pharmacovigilance practices (GVPs) and guidelines to prevent adverse drug reactions (ADRs) from licensed pharmaceutical medications harming people. Periodic Safety Update Reports (PSURs), which may give regulatory authorities an update on a drug's or medicinal product's global safety experience at specific time points after authorization, are one way to achieve these guidelines.

Farid A. Badria, Ph.D, D.Sc.
FAB-Lab,
Faculty of Pharmacy,
Pharmacognosy Department,
Mansoura University,
Mansoura, Egypt

Section 1

Innovation and Applications of AI Pharmacovigilance

Chapter 1

Optimizing Pharmacovigilance in an Era of Accelerating Innovation

Farid A. Badria and Abdullah A. Elgazar

Abstract

Pharmacovigilance involves detecting, assessing, understanding, and preventing adverse drug effects. The field aims to systematically monitor medicines and promote their safe, effective use. However, pharmacovigilance faces challenges such as fragmented systems and passive reporting. As the discipline advances, priorities now include centralizing data analysis, applying technologies like *AI* for safety signals, leveraging real-world data, implementing proactive risk planning, and increasing patient engagement. Recent advancements have emphasized the role of *machine learning* in identifying adverse drug reactions (ADRs), predicting drug-drug interactions, and enhancing personalized care. *Big Data* and *cloud computing* also play critical roles in facilitating the efficient analysis of massive healthcare datasets, contributing to earlier safety signal detection. Moreover, the emerging application of *blockchain technology* promises to revolutionize drug traceability, data security, and real-time reporting, thus improving drug safety monitoring. The COVID-19 pandemic revealed the need for robust systems that can enable rapid responses to emerging safety issues around epidemic treatments and vaccines. The next era of pharmacovigilance seeks to transform monitoring to improve patient outcomes worldwide. However, thoughtful implementation, focused on ethics, validity, and equity, is critical. The aim of this chapter is to provide perspectives on optimizing pharmacovigilance practices in an evolving landscape, integrating cutting-edge technologies to better safeguard patients.

Keywords: adverse drug effects, real-world data, artificial intelligence, big data, *blockchain technology*, proactive surveillance, patient engagement

1. Introduction

Pharmacovigilance is the process of monitoring, evaluating, and mitigating the potential risks associated with medicines and vaccines. Its critical role in ensuring patient safety cannot be overstated, as the history of drug development is marked by numerous instances where inadequate safety monitoring led to devastating consequences [1, 2]. One of the most infamous examples is the thalidomide tragedy, where the use of the drug thalidomide during pregnancy caused severe birth defects in thousands of children born in the late 1950s and early 1960s. This catastrophic event underscored the dire need for robust pharmacovigilance systems to detect adverse drug reactions before they cause widespread harm [3, 4].

The importance of pharmacovigilance extends beyond the initial approval process, as post-marketing surveillance is crucial for identifying rare or long-term side effects that may not have been apparent during clinical trials. The withdrawal of major blockbuster drugs from the market due to safety concerns further emphasizes the significance of continuous monitoring. For instance, the anti-inflammatory drug Vioxx (rofecoxib) was withdrawn in 2004 after being linked to an increased risk of heart attacks and strokes, while the diabetes medication Avandia (rosiglitazone) was severely restricted in 2010 due to its association with cardiovascular events [5, 6].

The thalidomide tragedy and the withdrawal of blockbuster drugs like Vioxx and Avandia serve as sobering reminders of the grave consequences that can arise when drug safety is compromised. These events have galvanized the pharmaceutical industry, regulatory agencies, and healthcare professionals to prioritize pharmacovigilance as a critical safeguard against potential harm to patients. The implementation of rigorous monitoring systems, prompt risk communication, and regulatory oversight have become paramount in the pursuit of delivering safe and effective medical treatments.

Furthermore, the COVID-19 pandemic has brought the importance of pharmacovigilance into sharp focus, as the rapid development and global distribution of vaccines and therapies necessitated robust safety monitoring mechanisms. The unprecedented scale of vaccination campaigns and the urgency to identify and mitigate potential adverse effects highlighted the indispensable role of pharmacovigilance in public health emergencies [7].

By exploring the fundamental principles, emerging technologies, global collaboration efforts, and future directions of pharmacovigilance, this chapter explores the critical role of pharmacovigilance in ensuring patient safety, the evolving technologies shaping the field, and its application across diverse areas of healthcare. The key themes covered include the fundamentals of pharmacovigilance, emerging technologies and data sources, global collaboration and regulatory frameworks, and the future of pharmacovigilance in precision medicine and specialized therapeutic areas. By exploring these topics, this chapter aims to underscore the vital function of pharmacovigilance in protecting public health and highlight the ongoing efforts to enhance its effectiveness in the face of rapid medical advancements.

2. The fundamentals of pharmacovigilance

Pharmacovigilance is an extremely important factor in ensuring that medicines are both safe and effective. Aspects such as the identification, evaluation, comprehension, and prevention of side effects or any other issues that are associated with medicines or vaccines are included in this process. So, it is a process that helps identify potential hazards and take appropriate measures, such as issuing safety alerts and implementing regulatory changes to safeguard patients. This is accomplished by monitoring and analyzing data on adverse pharmacological effects brought about by medications [8].

Pharmacovigilance can greatly benefit from the data that is provided by electronic health records (EHRs), enabling medical personnel to access comprehensive patient information, including medication history and adverse events, for more precise safety monitoring. Real-time monitoring systems enable continuous drug safety monitoring, facilitating the prompt detection of safety signals and ensuring timely responses to emerging risks. These systems make use of automated algorithms to analyze data from a variety of sources, including electronic medical records, social media, and healthcare databases [9].

After a drug or vaccine is approved for commercial use, pharmacovigilance plays a crucial role in monitoring its safety and efficacy in real-world settings. This process involves collecting and analyzing data from various sources, including spontaneous reports from healthcare professionals, patients, and pharmaceutical companies, as well as data from clinical studies and observational studies. For instance, the identification of rare or long-term adverse effects, such as the increased risk of heart attacks associated with certain pain medications (e.g., Rofecoxib), or the potential link between certain antidepressants and suicidal thoughts in adolescents, was facilitated by pharmacovigilance activities [10, 11].

Moreover, pharmacovigilance employs statistical and data mining techniques to identify potential safety signals, which are indications of new or previously unrecognized adverse drug reactions (ADRs). These signals can arise from various sources, including spontaneous reports, clinical trials, or observational studies. For example, the WHO Global Individual Case Safety Report (ICSR) database, VigiBase, contains over 20 million case reports of suspected ADRs from over 130 countries. Automated signal detection algorithms analyze this data to identify potential safety signals, which are then further investigated and evaluated by pharmacovigilance experts [9, 12].

Also, pharmacovigilance plays a crucial role in risk management, which involves identifying, assessing, and mitigating the risks associated with a particular drug or vaccine. This process involves developing and implementing risk minimization strategies, such as updating product labeling, issuing safety communications, or implementing risk evaluation and mitigation strategies (REMS) to ensure the safe use of the product. This could be applied in the case of immunosuppressant drugs to include measures to educate healthcare professionals and patients about the increased risk of infections and malignancies, as well as the need for regular monitoring [13].

Hence, pharmacovigilance data and findings are essential for regulatory authorities, such as the U.S. Food and Drug Administration (FDA) and the European Medicines Agency (EMA), in making informed decisions regarding drug approval, labeling, and post-marketing surveillance requirements. These agencies rely on pharmacovigilance data to identify potential safety concerns, issue safety alerts, and implement regulatory actions, such as product recalls or restrictions, when necessary [14]. For example, in 2020, the FDA issued a safety communication warning about the potential increased risk of heart rhythm problems associated with the use of certain antiarrhythmic drugs, such as amiodarone and sotalol, based on pharmacovigilance data and analysis [15, 16]. By continuously monitoring and evaluating the safety profile of drugs and vaccines, pharmacovigilance plays a vital role in safeguarding public health, reducing the burden of adverse drug reactions, and ensuring that the benefits of medicinal products outweigh their potential risks.

Table 1 summarize activities that would allow pharmacovigilance to improve drug safety.

Activity	Impact on drug safety
Early detection of safety signals	Pharmacovigilance activities enable the early detection of potential safety issues, allowing for timely interventions and risk mitigation strategies to protect patient safety.
Continuous monitoring	Throughout the product lifecycle ensures that any emerging safety concerns are promptly identified and addressed, reducing the risk of adverse events and improving patient outcomes.
Risk minimization	By implementing risk minimization strategies, such as updating product labeling, issuing safety communications, or implementing REMS, pharmacovigilance helps mitigate the risks associated with drug use and promotes safer prescribing and administration practices.
Regulatory decision-making	Pharmacovigilance data and analysis inform regulatory decisions regarding product approval, labeling, and post-marketing surveillance requirements, ensuring that only safe and effective drugs are available on the market and that appropriate measures are in place to monitor and address potential safety concerns.
Public trust and confidence	Robust pharmacovigilance activities and transparent communication of safety information help build public trust and confidence in the pharmaceutical industry and regulatory authorities, promoting adherence to treatment regimens and improving overall public health outcomes.

Table 1.
Impact of pharmacovigilance activity on improving drug safety.

3. Emerging technologies and data sources in pharmacovigilance

As a result of the rapid pace of innovation in the healthcare industry, the field of pharmacovigilance is undergoing rapid change. Artificial intelligence (AI), machine learning, and real-time monitoring systems are examples of cutting-edge technologies that are bringing about a revolution in the detection and evaluation of adverse medication effects. In the field of pharmacovigilance, the application of artificial intelligence (AI) techniques, such as natural language processing and machine learning, has the potential to improve indicator detection. With the use of artificial intelligence algorithms, enormous amounts of data may be analyzed, and patterns that may suggest potential hazardous pharmacological effects can be identified [17].

It is possible to utilize algorithms that are based on machine learning to evaluate the risk associated with particular medications or drug combinations. The identification of factors that lead to higher risk can be accomplished using machine learning models through the analysis of data on adverse events and patient characteristics. In the field of pharmacovigilance, data mining tools have the ability to unearth previously concealed patterns and relationships. The use of data mining techniques allows for the identification of previously undiscovered correlations between medications and adverse occurrences [18, 19].

The various social media platforms offer a lot of information that can be utilized for the purpose of pharmacovigilance. Through the use of social media, patients frequently report adverse occurrences and share their experiences, which provides vital insights into the safety of medications. Additionally, wearable devices like smartwatches and fitness trackers play a crucial role in providing real-time monitoring of patient health metrics, enabling early detection of adverse events, and enhancing patient safety in pharmacovigilance [20–22].

AI can help transform pharmacovigilance from being primarily reactive to becoming more proactive in identifying and mitigating potential safety issues. In this context, an AI system could analyze data from preclinical animal studies and early-phase clinical trials to predict the likelihood of specific adverse events occurring in later-phase trials or post-marketing surveillance. This predictive capability allows for proactive risk mitigation strategies and targeted monitoring plans [20, 23].

Furthermore, AI can help stratify patient populations based on their risk profiles for specific adverse events. By identifying high-risk subgroups, pharmacovigilance efforts can be focused on these populations, enabling proactive monitoring and targeted risk minimization interventions. Additionally, this information could guide the enrichment of clinical trials with appropriate patient populations and inform tailored risk management plans [24].

Interestingly, AI systems could continuously monitor and analyze data on a drug's efficacy, safety, and real-world usage patterns. If the system detects a shift in the benefit-risk profile, it could alert pharmacovigilance teams to consider proactive actions, such as updating product labeling, implementing risk minimization measures, or potentially reevaluating the drug's approval status. Finally, AI can simulate various scenarios and model the potential impact of different risk mitigation strategies. This can help pharmacovigilance teams proactively plan and prepare for potential safety issues, enabling more effective and timely responses [22].

In this context, a recent systematic review showed that the most common uses of AI, particularly machine learning, in pharmacovigilance included the identification of adverse drug events (ADEs) and adverse drug reactions (ADRs) (57.6% of studies), processing safety reports (21.2%), and extracting or predicting drug-drug interactions (7.6%). Other applications included identifying high-risk populations for drug toxicity and guiding personalized care (7.6%), predicting side effects (3.0%), simulating clinical trials (1.5%), and integrating prediction uncertainties into diagnostic classifiers to enhance patient safety (1.5%) [25].

Artificial Intelligence (AI) capabilities, when applied to Big Data analysis, enable more efficient predictions of potential adverse drug effects. This approach has successfully revealed new connections between diseases and risk factors. In the pharmaceutical development lifecycle, Big Data analysis has found critical applications in genomics, clinical monitoring, and pharmacovigilance. Technologies like Hadoop facilitate the management of large datasets, allowing researchers to derive insights from vast amounts of biomedical data. Cloud computing serves as a versatile repository for these large datasets, offering scalable and efficient storage and processing. This makes it feasible to analyze extensive healthcare databases, projected to reach 10 terabytes, containing detailed medical records and clinical data [26].

Furthermore, cloud computing supports advanced statistical algorithms like MapReduce and Hadoop, enabling real-time analytics on heterogeneous patient data. Such technological advancements are crucial for initiatives like PCORnet, which aims to create a comprehensive repository of medical information from millions of Americans. By integrating these technologies, the pharmaceutical industry can perform more comprehensive and efficient pharmacovigilance, potentially leading to earlier detection of drug safety issues and more effective risk management, ultimately resulting in safer and more effective medications [27].

By leveraging AI's predictive capabilities, risk stratification, continuous monitoring, and scenario planning, pharmacovigilance can transition from a primarily reactive approach to a more proactive, anticipatory model. This shift allows for earlier identification of potential safety issues, targeted risk mitigation strategies, and more efficient allocation of resources, ultimately enhancing patient safety and optimizing the benefit-risk profiles of pharmaceutical products [28]. **Table 2** summarizes the main application of AI in pharmacovigilance.

Pharmacovigilance elements	Artificial intelligence application
Predictive signal detection	Identify potential safety signals before actual adverse event reports, enabling proactive risk mitigation strategies and targeted monitoring plans.
Risk stratification and patient enrichment	Stratify patient populations based on risk profiles for specific adverse events, allowing proactive monitoring and targeted interventions for high-risk subgroups.
Continuous benefit-risk evaluation	Continuously evaluate the benefit-risk profile of drugs by integrating data from multiple sources, enabling proactive adjustments to risk management strategies, label updates, or other interventions.
Simulation and scenario planning	Simulate various scenarios and model the potential impact of different risk mitigation strategies, allowing for proactive contingency planning and effective response preparedness.
Clinical data repository and Big Data bases	Analyze large volumes of data from various sources (reports, literature, social media, EHRs) to detect patterns and signals, enabling earlier detection and faster response times using natural language processing (NLP) and machine learning (ML).
Case prioritization and triage	Prioritize and triage incoming adverse event reports based on severity and risk, streamlining the process and ensuring prompt attention to high-risk cases.
Causality assessment	Evaluate the potential causal relationship between a drug and an adverse event, providing insights into the likelihood of causation for further investigation.
Literature monitoring	Continuously monitor and analyze the latest scientific literature, identifying emerging safety signals or new information relevant to a drug's safety profile.

Table 2.
Application of artificial intelligence in optimization of pharmacovigilance activities.

4. Global collaboration and regulatory frameworks

In order to make pharmacovigilance more effective, collaboration with regulatory agencies is absolutely necessary. By exchanging information and knowledge, pharmacovigilance systems are able to gain access to a more comprehensive perspective and guarantee that safety requirements are maintained consistently. Networks for global pharmacovigilance, such as the World Health Organization's Program for International Drug Monitoring, are extremely important in the process of fostering pharmacovigilance on a global scale. For pharmacovigilance to be effective, it is necessary for numerous stakeholders, such as healthcare professionals, researchers, patients, and representatives from the industry, to work together and share their information [28, 29].

This was best shown in 2010 when a rare but serious adverse event (progressive multifocal leukoencephalopathy) associated with the multiple sclerosis drug Natalizumab was first detected in the United States. Through global collaboration and data sharing via platforms like VigiBase, regulatory authorities and pharmaceutical companies worldwide were promptly alerted, enabling coordinated monitoring, risk assessment, and implementation of risk minimization measures globally [29, 30]. Also, in 2017, the European Medicines Agency (EMA) and the U.S. Food and Drug Administration (FDA) collaborated closely to investigate and address safety concerns related to gadolinium-based contrast agents used in MRI scans. This coordinated effort led to simultaneous label updates and risk communication strategies across multiple regions, ensuring consistent messaging and risk minimization measures for patients globally [31–33].

Global collaboration would allow the experience transfer of Good Pharmacovigilance Practices (GVP) guidelines to the newly established pharmacovigilance centers. GVPs are intended to standardize the collection, analysis, and reporting of adverse medication reactions, ensuring consistency and regulatory compliance in pharmacovigilance activities. Audits of pharmacovigilance are absolutely necessary in order to evaluate the efficiency and conformity of pharmacovigilance systems. Pharmacovigilance systems must comply with regulatory reporting requirements for adverse events and safety signals to ensure patient safety and regulatory adherence which would strengthen and development of global collaboration. **Table 3** summarizes GVP.

Because of the rapid improvements in pharmacovigilance technology and methods, regulatory frameworks need to be able to keep up with these changes. While preserving the safety of patients and the security of their data, it is essential to modify legislation so that they can accept developing technologies, such as artificial intelligence and evidence from the real-world. A number of ethical and legal challenges are brought up by pharmacovigilance, including patient privacy, data protection, and seeking informed permission. In order to ensure that pharmacovigilance processes comply with ethical values and legal criteria, it is essential to address these problems and make sure that regulations are followed [34, 35].

In this context, Blockchain technology offers significant potential to revolutionize pharmacovigilance practices, enhancing drug safety monitoring and reporting. By leveraging its decentralized and tamper-proof nature, blockchain ensures data

Aspect	Description
Scope and applicability	• Applies to marketing authorization holders (MAHs), European Medicines Agency (EMA), and medicines regulatory authorities in EU Member States. Covers centrally authorized medicines and those authorized at the national level
Modules and topics	• Divided into modules, each covering a specific aspect of pharmacovigilance. Modules address processes such as risk management, signal detection, periodic safety update reports, post-authorization safety studies, etc.
Revision and review	• Regularly reviewed to ensure they remain up to date and relevant to revision based on emerging scientific knowledge, regulatory changes, and stakeholder feedback
Signal detection and assessment	• Provides guidance on safety signal identification and interpretation. Outlines principles and methodologies for assessing potential risks associated with medicines based on observational data and other sources
Pharmacovigilance plan development	• Offers guidance on the development of pharmacovigilance plans. Plans outline strategies and activities MAHs should undertake to monitor product safety throughout their lifecycle
Compliance and inspections	• Compliance with GVP guidelines is essential for MAHs and other stakeholders. Authorities conduct inspections to assess compliance with GVP requirements and ensure proper implementation of pharmacovigilance systems
Pharmacovigilance plan development	• Offers guidance on the development of pharmacovigilance plans. Plans outline strategies and activities MAHs should undertake to monitor product safety throughout their lifecycle
Compliance and inspections	• Compliance with GVP guidelines is essential for MAHs and other stakeholders. Regulatory authorities conduct inspections to assess compliance with GVP requirements and ensure proper implementation of pharmacovigilance systems

Table 3.
Good pharmacovigilance practices.

integrity and security for adverse event reports and safety data [36]. It improves drug traceability throughout the supply chain, enabling precise tracking of origins and batch-specific adverse reactions [37].

The technology facilitates real-time ADR reporting, empowering healthcare professionals and patients to contribute directly to a secure network, thus accelerating safety signal identification. Blockchain also addresses patient privacy concerns by allowing individuals to control their health data sharing while maintaining anonymity. Furthermore, it promotes collaboration among stakeholders by enabling secure data sharing, and its smart contract capabilities can automate critical pharmacovigilance processes, such as safety alerts and compensation management. These features collectively contribute to a more robust, efficient, and transparent system for ensuring pharmaceutical safety [38]. For example, a recent report from Kenya showed that applying blockchain technology could help the patient to patients to determine the legitimacy of their purchased drugs, thereby helping to reduce and potentially eradicate the problem of counterfeit medications in the market [39].

While this field is very promising, the success of its implementation requires careful consideration of several factors, such as the extent of access, interoperability, and scalability of healthcare blockchains following the implementation of various strategies and frameworks. Additionally, the impact of computational performance and the costs and benefits of using blockchain systems [40].

5. The COVID-19 pandemic and pharmacovigilance

The COVID-19 pandemic has highlighted the critical importance of pharmacovigilance. It has become more important to have comprehensive pharmacovigilance systems in place in order to guarantee the safe and effective utilization of COVID-19 vaccines and therapies, which have been rapidly developed and implemented. During the pandemic, pharmacovigilance was an extremely important factor in the early detection and evaluation of probable adverse effects that were connected with COVID-19 vaccinations and medicines. The vast amount of data that was created from the global vaccination campaigns was one of the most significant obstacles that COVID-19 pharmacovigilance needed to overcome. When it came to COVID-19 pharmacovigilance, collaboration and information sharing among stakeholders, such as regulatory authorities, healthcare practitioners, and pharmaceutical corporations, were absolutely necessary [41].

For example, The Inserm Safety Department encountered significant hurdles in managing safety data during a large-scale European clinical trial investigating repurposed and investigational drugs for COVID-19 treatment. The department was overwhelmed with a high volume of safety reports, handling 585 initial serious adverse event (SAE) notifications and 396 follow-up reports. Data quality issues further compounded the challenges, as more than 500 queries were sent to investigators due to missing or incoherent information on the SAE forms, making the evaluation and assessment of reported SAEs difficult [42].

Moreover, delays in accurately completing SAE forms, coupled with the need for real-time medical analysis, posed major obstacles in promptly identifying potential safety signals from the trial data. These challenges underscored the substantial workload, data quality concerns, and timing issues faced by the pharmacovigilance team, potentially impacting their ability to efficiently detect and respond to safety signals during this critical pandemic-related clinical research [43, 44].

A study involving hospital pharmacists in France highlighted their crucial role in enhancing drug management for COVID-19 patients. The pharmacists conducted 575 pharmaceutical interventions across 1483 hospitalized patients, including 444 with COVID-19, identifying issues such as overdoses, untreated indications, and drug-drug interactions. Notably, patients with COVID-19 experienced significantly more adverse medication events, with 73.3% involving disease-specific therapies. Pharmacovigilance reports were performed for a substantial portion of patients treated with hydroxychloroquine (25%) and lopinavir/ritonavir (33%), underscoring the importance of safety monitoring for these COVID-19 treatments. The study highlights the invaluable contribution of hospital pharmacists in managing COVID-19 patients' medication regimens, particularly in the context of evolving therapies and vaccine implementation, where their expertise can help optimize drug safety and efficacy [45].

In addition, the COVID-19 pandemic brought to light the significance of actively involving patients and the general public in pharmacovigilance activities. Digital technologies and social media platforms were deployed for the purpose of facilitating adverse event reporting and gathering patient experiences. More importantly, COVID-19 pharmacovigilance highlighted the importance of having comprehensive post-marketing monitoring systems to monitor the long-term safety of medicines and vaccines [46, 47].

6. The role of pharmacovigilance in the integration of traditional medicine in healthcare systems

Integrating herbal and traditional medicines into mainstream healthcare systems presents a significant challenge in identifying potential adverse effects that may arise from their use [48, 49]. A major obstacle is the general perception that traditional remedies are safe, leading patients not to disclose their use to healthcare professionals. This lack of communication can increase the risk of adverse drug reactions (ADRs) or drug-herb interactions when traditional medicines are used concomitantly with conventional medications [50].

To successfully incorporate traditional medicine into pharmacovigilance systems, it is crucial for practitioners of traditional medicine and experts in pharmacovigilance to collaborate and share their knowledge. Patient education by traditional practitioners and their ability to anticipate potential adverse effects require involving them in pharmacovigilance activities and providing appropriate training [51, 52].

Pharmacovigilance efforts have played a vital role in identifying and mitigating risks associated with the concomitant use of traditional medicines and conventional drugs. For instance, post-marketing surveillance and case reports revealed that St. John's Wort, a popular herbal supplement, can induce liver enzymes responsible for metabolizing various medications. This interaction can lead to decreased drug efficacy or increased risk of adverse events. Consequently, regulatory agencies issued safety communications and label updates, warning about the potential for reduced therapeutic effects when St. John's Wort is taken with medications like oral contraceptives, antiretrovirals, or certain cancer therapies [53, 54].

Another example involves the use of Traditional Chinese Medicine (TCM) in patients undergoing conventional cancer treatments. Pharmacovigilance studies identified potential interactions between specific TCM herbal formulations and chemotherapeutic agents, leading to increased toxicity or reduced efficacy of the cancer treatments. In response, healthcare authorities provided guidance on safe concomitant use, recommending that patients consult with their oncologists before taking any TCM products during cancer therapy to prevent potential ADRs or compromised treatment outcomes [55].

In some cases, pharmacovigilance data has prompted regulatory actions to mitigate risks. Reports of severe liver injury and other adverse events associated with the concurrent use of certain dietary supplements and prescription medications led the United States Food and Drug Administration (FDA) to issue warnings and consider regulatory actions, such as product recalls or stricter labeling requirements, to promote safer use and prevent harm to patients [56, 57].

Furthermore, pharmacovigilance efforts have facilitated risk communication and awareness campaigns. In regions where traditional medicine practices are widespread, pharmacovigilance authorities have collaborated with local communities and traditional healers to educate patients and healthcare providers about potential drug-herb interactions and safe practices when combining traditional and conventional therapies [58, 59].

By continuously monitoring, assessing, and communicating the risks associated with the concurrent use of traditional medicines and conventional drugs, pharmacovigilance plays a vital role in promoting safer and more informed use of these therapies, ultimately contributing to improved patient safety and better treatment outcomes.

7. The future of pharmacovigilance: Precision medicine and specialized areas

The application of tailored therapies that are determined by the features of the individual patient is what is meant by the term "precision medicine." Identifying safety profiles that are unique to these targeted medicines ought to be the primary emphasis of pharmacovigilance in the future. An evaluation of the influence that pharmacogenomic variability has on the efficacy and safety of drugs should be part of pharmacovigilance.

Gene and cell therapies have their own distinct set of safety issues, which necessitate the implementation of specialist pharmacovigilance assessments. The mechanisms of action that are involved in these therapies are frequently novel, and they have the potential to have long-term consequences. In order to ensure that gene and cell therapies are safe throughout their entire lifecycle, pharmacovigilance needs to create particular ways to monitor their safety. Hence, a new term called precision pharmacovigilance emerged [60, 61].

In this approach, advancements in personalized medicine, genomics, and other molecular technologies enhance the safety monitoring and risk management of pharmaceutical products. It involves tailoring pharmacovigilance activities to specific patient subgroups or individuals based on their genetic, clinical, and environmental characteristics. For instance, patients carrying specific human leukocyte antigen (HLA) alleles have been found to be at a significantly higher risk for developing severe cutaneous adverse reactions, such as Stevens-Johnson syndrome or toxic epidermal necrolysis, when exposed to certain drugs like carbamazepine or abacavir [62, 63].

By identifying these genetic risk factors, precision pharmacovigilance enables targeted safety monitoring and preemptive risk mitigation strategies, such as genetic screening or alternative treatment options, for high-risk patient populations. This personalized approach to safety surveillance can significantly improve the benefit-risk profile of medications and enhance patient safety outcomes.

8. Conclusion

In this era of rapid technological advancement, optimizing pharmacovigilance processes is essential. By embracing modern data-gathering methods, leveraging emerging technologies, boosting collaboration, and maintaining regulatory compliance, pharmacovigilance can enhance the effectiveness of monitoring adverse drug effects and improve patient safety. *The integration of AI and machine learning enables faster detection of adverse drug events and adverse drug reactions, helping identify high-risk populations and predict side effects more accurately. Furthermore, Big Data and cloud computing facilitate the analysis of vast healthcare datasets, which is crucial for real-time safety monitoring.*

In order to ensure the safety of drugs, it is necessary to provide patients with information that is both understandable and easily available. Patients ought to have access to detailed information regarding the advantages and disadvantages of the medications they take, as well as instructions on how to report anything that goes wrong with their medications. Effective risk communication strategies ought to be the top priority for pharmacovigilance, and they should emphasize their development and execution. **Figure 1** represents how pharmacovigilance could be involved in health care to achieve better outcomes.

To ensure drug safety, it is necessary to provide patients with understandable and easily accessible information. Patients should have access to detailed insights into the risks and benefits of their medications, along with clear instructions on how to report adverse reactions. Effective risk communication strategies must be a priority, with a focus on their development and implementation. *Blockchain technology, with its decentralized and tamper-proof nature, promises significant enhancements in drug traceability and data security, helping prevent counterfeit medications and ensuring real-time ADR reporting.*

In the future of pharmacovigilance, proactive and tailored approaches that put the patient's well-being first will be the most important components. Pharmacovigilance has the potential to play a significant role in patient protection if it continues to adapt to the rapidly evolving technological landscape. *By leveraging advanced technologies like AI, Big Data analytics, and blockchain, while also maintaining a focus on patient-centric care and effective communication, pharmacovigilance can contribute significantly to optimizing patient outcomes and fostering a culture of medication safety across the healthcare landscape.*

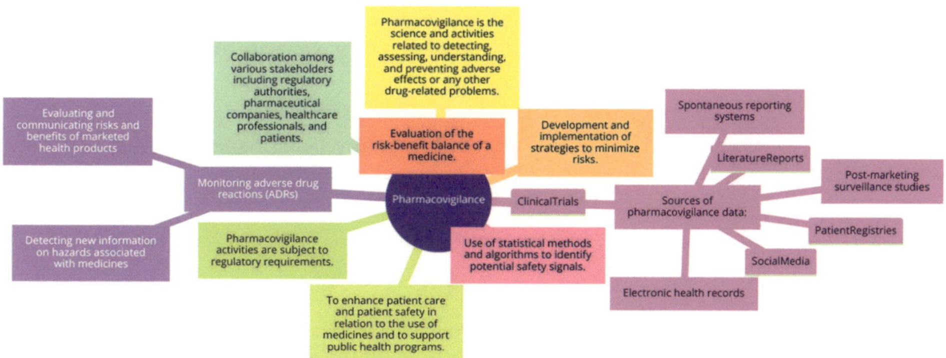

Figure 1.
Mind map outlines the core elements of pharmacovigilance, including its definition, purpose, key activities, data sources, and risk management strategies.

Acknowledgements

The authors acknowledge the use of Chat GPT for language polishing of the manuscript.

Conflict of interest

The authors declare no conflict of interest.

Author details

Farid A. Badria[1]* and Abdullah A. Elgazar[2]

1 Department of Pharmacognosy, Faculty of Pharmacy, Mansoura University, Mansoura, Egypt

2 Department of Pharmacognosy, Faculty of Pharmacy, Kafrelsheikh University, Kafrelsheikh, Egypt

*Address all correspondence to: faridbadria@gmail.com

IntechOpen

© 2024 The Author(s). Licensee IntechOpen. This chapter is distributed under the terms of the Creative Commons Attribution License (http://creativecommons.org/licenses/by/4.0), which permits unrestricted use, distribution, and reproduction in any medium, provided the original work is properly cited.

References

[1] Beninger P. Pharmacovigilance: An overview. Clinical Therapeutics. 2018;**40**:1991-2004

[2] Meyboom RHB, Egberts ACG, Gribnau FWJ, Hekster YA. Pharmacovigilance in perspective. Drug Safety. 1999;**21**:429-447

[3] Rehman W, Arfons LM, Lazarus HM. The rise, fall and subsequent triumph of thalidomide: Lessons learned in drug development. Therapeutic Advances in Hematology. 2011;**2**:291-308

[4] Javid M, Nandave M, Kumar A. History of pharmacovigilance. In: Pharmacovigilance Essentials: Advances, Challenges and Global Perspectives. Berlin, Germany: Springer Nature; 2024. pp. 19-53

[5] Barry AR, Koshman SL, Pearson GJ. Adverse drug reactions: The importance of maintaining pharmacovigilance. Canadian Pharmacists Journal/ Revue des Pharmaciens du Canada. 2014;**147**:233-238

[6] Gale EAM. Collateral damage: The conundrum of drug safety. Diabetologia. 2009;**52**:1975-1982

[7] Dutta S, Ambwani S, Mishra G, Lal HI, Ram K, Kumar T. Pharmacovigilance in the era of Covid-19: A concise review of the current scenario, implications, and challenges. International Journal of Applied Pharmaceutics. 2021;**13**:1-4

[8] Van Grootheest AC, Richesson RL. Pharmacovigilance. In: Clinical Research Informatics. Berlin, Germany: Springer; 2012. pp. 367-387

[9] Lee J. A discussion about pharmacovigilance study methods. Journal of Korean Medical Science. 2024;**39**

[10] Devi R, Devi A, Kumar S, Jeet K, Sharma T, Sharma S, et al. Good clinical practice in pharmacovigilance. International Journal of Advanced Research. 2022;**10**(4):428-433

[11] Rogers A, Grieve K, MacDonald TM, Nishioka S. COX-2 inhibitors: Communication of accumulating risk evidence and a product withdrawal. In: Communicating about Risks and Safe Use of Medicines: Real Life and Applied Research. Berlin, Germany: Springer Nature; 2020. pp. 131-146

[12] Bihan K, Lebrun-Vignes B, Funck-Brentano C, Salem J-E. Uses of pharmacovigilance databases: An overview. Thérapie. 2020;**75**:591-598

[13] Tiwari P, Deshwal PR. Pharmacovigilance. In: Drug Discovery and Development: From Targets and Molecules to Medicines. Germany: Springer; 2021. pp. 435-449

[14] Mansuri A, Zaman TU. Pharmacovigilance: A necessary tool for drug safety monitoring globally. Journal of Drug Delivery and Therapeutics. 2024;**14**:96-103

[15] Lenhoff H. Risks and risk monitoring in Sotalol therapy for atrial fibrillation. Karolinska Institutet (Sweden). 2023. pp. 22-23

[16] Wang F, Zhou B, Sun H, Wu X. Proarrhythmia associated with antiarrhythmic drugs: A comprehensive disproportionality analysis of the FDA adverse event reporting system. Frontiers in Pharmacology. 2023;**14**:1170039

[17] Ibara MA, Richesson RL. Back to the future: The evolution of pharmacovigilance in the age of digital

healthcare. In: Clinical Research Informatics. Berlin, Germany: Springer Nature; 2023. pp. 455-471

[18] Pilipiec P, Liwicki M, Bota A. Using machine learning for pharmacovigilance: A systematic review. Pharmaceutics. 2022;**14**:266

[19] Kompa B, Hakim JB, Palepu A, Kompa KG, Smith M, Bain PA, et al. Artificial intelligence based on machine learning in pharmacovigilance: A scoping review. Drug Safety. 2022;**45**:477-491

[20] Hauben M. Artificial intelligence and data mining for the pharmacovigilance of drug–drug interactions. Clinical Therapeutics. 2023;**45**:117-133

[21] Dhingra P, Gayathri N, Kumar SR, Singanamalla V, Ramesh C, Balamurugan B. Internet of Things–based pharmaceutics data analysis. In: Emergence of Pharmaceutical Industry Growth with Industrial IoT Approach. Berlin, Germany: Springer Nature; 2020. pp. 85-131

[22] Nadar S, Devi A, Jain R, Al-Turjman F. Use of artificial intelligence in pharmacovigilance for social media network. In: Leveraging Artificial Intelligence in Global Epidemics. Berlin, Germany: Springer Nature; 2021. pp. 239-259

[23] Salvo F, Micallef J, Lahouegue A, Chouchana L, Létinier L, Faillie J-L, et al. Will the future of pharmacovigilance be more automated? Expert Opinion on Drug Safety. 2023;**22**:541-548

[24] Kalaiselvan V, Sharma A, Gupta SK. "Feasibility test and application of AI in healthcare"—With special emphasis in clinical, pharmacovigilance, and regulatory practices. Health and Technology. 2021;**11**:1-15

[25] Salas M, Petracek J, Yalamanchili P, Aimer O, Kasthuril D, Dhingra S, et al. The use of artificial intelligence in pharmacovigilance: A systematic review of the literature. Pharmaceutical Medicine. 2022;**36**:295-306

[26] Schultz T. Turning healthcare challenges into big data opportunities: A use-case review across the pharmaceutical development lifecycle. Bulletin of the American Society for Information Science and Technology. 2013;**39**:34-40

[27] Celi LA, Moseley E, Moses C, Ryan P, Somai M, Stone D, et al. From pharmacovigilance to clinical care optimization. Big Data. 2014;**2**:134-141

[28] Nord M, Ysander M, Sullivan T, Patel M. Practical considerations for creating a strategic and proactive clinical safety and pharmacovigilance organization for the future. International Journal of Risk & Safety in Medicine. 2021;**32**:243-258

[29] Isah A, Opadeyi A, Cobelens F, Tumwijukye H. The standalone pharmacovigilance policy: A tool for engagement and collaboration of stakeholders in the pharmacovigilance system in resource limited settings. Drug Safety. 2021;**44**:1450-1451

[30] Peyro-Saint-Paul L, Fedrizzi S, Defer G. Drug safety in multiple sclerosis: From reporting to signal detection and benefit-risk management. Revue Neurologique. 2021;**177**:582-588

[31] Di Grezia G, Gatta G, Iannaccone T. Contrast media pharmacovigilance in diagnostic imaging: A tool to enhance. Pharmacology. 2021;**1**:158-165

[32] Shahid I, Joseph A, Lancelot E. Use of real-life safety data from international pharmacovigilance databases to assess the importance of symptoms associated with gadolinium exposure. Investigative Radiology. 2022;**57**:664-673

[33] Cooper D, Platt RW, van Hunsel F, Davies M, Yeomans A, Lane S, et al. The international working group on new developments in pharmacovigilance: Advancing methods and communication in pharmacovigilance. Clinical Therapeutics. 2024;**46**(7):565-569

[34] Chinchilla K, Matos C, Hall V, van Hunsel F. Patient organizations' barriers in pharmacovigilance and strategies to stimulate their participation. Drug Safety. 2021;**44**:181-191

[35] Inácio P, Cavaco A, Airaksinen M. The value of patient reporting to the pharmacovigilance system: A systematic review. British Journal of Clinical Pharmacology. 2017;**83**:227-246

[36] Mokrova LP, Borodina MA, Goncharov VV, Popov SA, Kepa YN. Prospects for using blockchain technology in healthcare: Supply chain management. Entomology and Applied Science Letters. 2021;**8**:71-77

[37] Al-Worafi YM. Blockchain for drug safety. In: Technology for Drug Safety: Current Status and Future Developments. Berlin, Germany: Springer Nature; 2023. pp. 103-113

[38] Polshettiwar S, Mali S, Kamble N. Drug traceability using blockchain. In: Unleashing the Potentials of Blockchain Technology for Healthcare Industries. Amsterdam, The Netherlands: Elsevier; 2023. pp. 235-251

[39] Ogwel PT. Blockchain Enabled Drug Traceability Solution: A Case of Drug Counterfeiting in a Pharmaceutical Supply Chain. Doctoral dissertation, Strathmore University, Nairobi, Kenya; 2020

[40] Meinert E, Alturkistani A, Foley KA, Osama T, Car J, Majeed A, et al. Blockchain implementation in health care: Protocol for a systematic review. JMIR Research Protocols. 2019;**8**:e10994

[41] Mouliou DS, Dardiotis E. Current evidence in SARS-CoV-2 mRNA vaccines and post-vaccination adverse reports: Knowns and unknowns. Diagnostics. 2022;**12**(7):1555-1570

[42] Baudouin A, Guillemin M-D, Rioufol C, Ranchon F, Parat S. Pandémie à SARS-COV-2: Implication du pharmacien hospitalier dans la sécurisation de la prise en charge des patients. Annales Pharmaceutiques Françaises. 2023;**81**:900-908

[43] Delgado A, Stewart S, Urroz M, Rodríguez A, Borobia AM, Akatbach-Bousaid I, et al. Characterisation of drug-induced liver injury in patients with COVID-19 detected by a proactive pharmacovigilance program from laboratory signals. Journal of Clinical Medicine. 2021;**10**:4432-4448

[44] Manzano AO, Cordeiro FB, Garcia-Angulo A, Carvajal-Aldaz D, Centeno E, Vizcaíno MJ, et al. Pharmacovigilance of the COVID-19 Vaccine in Ecuador during the First and Second Doses of Vaccination Campaigns. Bethesda, Maryland, USA: ASPET; 2023

[45] Baudouin A, Guillemin M-D, Rioufol C, Ranchon F, Parat S. SARS-COV-2 pandemic: Involvement of the hospital pharmacist in securing patient care. Annales Pharmaceutiques Françaises. Vol. **81**. S0003-S4509

[46] Tuccori M, Convertino I, Ferraro S, Cappello E, Valdiserra G, Focosi D, et al. The impact of the COVID-19 "Infodemic" on drug-utilization behaviors: Implications for pharmacovigilance. Drug Safety. 2020;**43**:699-709

[47] Koss J, Bohnet-Joschko S. Social media mining of long-COVID self-medication reported by Reddit users: Feasibility study to support drug repurposing. JMIR Formative Research. 2022;**6**:e39582

[48] Badria FA, Elgazar AA. Utilization of selected natural products as complementary therapeutic approach for Obstructive Sleep Apnea (OSA) management: A literature review. Clinical Phytoscience. 2024;**10**:15

[49] Abass SA, Elgazar AA, El-Kholy SS, El-Refaiy AI, Nawaya RA, Bhat MA, et al. Unraveling the nephroprotective potential of papaverine against cisplatin toxicity through mitigating oxidative stress and inflammation: Insights from in silico, in vitro, and in vivo investigations. Molecules. 2024;**29**:1927

[50] Kumar P, Nandave M, Kumar A, Nandave D. Herbovigilance. In: Pharmacovigilance Essentials: Advances, Challenges and Global Perspectives. Berlin, Germany: Springer; 2024. pp. 243-267

[51] Rastogi S. Why and how? Addressing to the two most pertinent questions about pharmacovigilance in Ayurveda. International Journal of Ayurveda Research. 2011;**2**:48

[52] Kim M, Woo Y, Han C-h. Current status of the spontaneous reporting and classification/coding system for herbal and traditional medicine in pharmacovigilance. Integrative Medicine Research. 2021;**10**:100467

[53] Choudhury A, Singh PA, Bajwa N, Dash S, Bisht P. Pharmacovigilance of herbal medicines: Concerns and future prospects. Journal of Ethnopharmacology. 2023;**309**:116383

[54] Aronson JK. The historical development of pharmacovigilance for herbal medicines. In: Pharmacovigilance for Herbal and Traditional Medicines: Advances, Challenges and International Perspectives. Berlin, Germany: Springer; 2022. pp. 3-13

[55] Pochet S, Lechon A-S, Lescrainier C, De Vriese C, Mathieu V, Hamdani J, et al. Herb-anticancer drug interactions in real life based on VigiBase, the WHO global database. Scientific Reports. 2022;**12**:14178

[56] Wang J-b, Gao Y, Guo Y-m, Xiao X-h. Pharmacovigilance for herbal and traditional medicine-induced liver injury. In: Pharmacovigilance for Herbal and Traditional Medicines: Advances, Challenges and International Perspectives. Berlin, Germany: Springer; 2022. pp. 41-50

[57] Teschke R, Danan G. Causality assessment in pharmacovigilance for herbal medicines. In: Pharmacovigilance for Herbal and Traditional Medicines: Advances, Challenges and International Perspectives. Berlin, Germany: Springer; 2022. pp. 189-209

[58] Pervaiz AD, Nahida R, Shameem AR, Farooq AD, Shabir APD, Hussain IMT. Proactive pharmacovigilance of Unani drugs, prospects and challenges. Journal of Pharmacovigilance. 2020;**8**:285

[59] Barnes J. Advances in methods and techniques in pharmacovigilance for herbal and traditional medicines and other natural health products. In: Pharmacovigilance for Herbal and Traditional Medicines: Advances, Challenges and International Perspectives. Berlin, Germany: Springer; 2022. pp. 93-139

[60] Silva L, Pacheco T, Araújo E, Duarte RJ, Ribeiro-Vaz I, Ferreira-da-Silva R. Unveiling the future: Precision pharmacovigilance in the era of personalized medicine. International

Journal of Clinical Pharmacy. 2024;**60**:1-6

[61] Petitpain N, Antoine ML, Beurrier M, Micallef J, Fresse A. Pharmacovigilance of Gene Therapy Medicinal Products. Rare Disease and Orphan Drugs Journal. Los Angeles, California, USA: OAE. 2023;**2**:25

[62] Jantararoungtong T, Tempark T, Koomdee N, Medhasi S, Sukasem C. Genotyping HLA alleles to predict the development of severe cutaneous adverse drug reactions (SCARs): State-of-the-art. Expert Opinion on Drug Metabolism & Toxicology. 2021;**17**:1049-1064

[63] Tsukagoshi E, Tanaka Y, Saito Y. Implementation of pharmacogenomic information on Stevens-Johnson syndrome and toxic epidermal necrolysis. Frontiers in Medicine (Lausanne). 2021;**8**:644154

Chapter 2

Perspective Chapter: Application of Artificial Intelligence in Pharmacovigilance Practices

Mohamed Gamaleldin, Shaimaa Abdelhalim and Ivo Abraham

Abstract

Patient exposure to medication during drug therapy makes the need for pharmacovigilance an integral part of patient safety. It is also followed by how the medicine enter into market phases. Pharmacovigilance systems and post-market surveillance reports ensure that regulatory authorities could monitor and assess adverse drug reactions in real time. Through the progress and innovations in artificial intelligence, which is getting its applications widely implemented in several healthcare domains these days, this has brought systems that could give the results quickly with high-level accuracy compared to those of humans. These systems are being employed to reduce adverse drug reactions (ADR), pick up safety signals swiftly, and serve as a directional tool to enable qualified entities of stakeholders, regulatory authorities, and pharmaceutical companies for the subsequent informed decision making. Artificial intelligence (AI) systems are changing healthcare and pharmaceuticals for a variety of reasons, including the speed at which they can be quickly advanced. Healthcare providers, regulatory agencies, and drug companies need to employ such systems in their pharmacovigilance practices. This chapter covers the application of artificial intelligence in pharmacovigilance systems and provides overview on integration of pharmacovigilance with AI for dummies. This chapter reviews the advantages and drawbacks of using AI in pharmacovigilance, creating regulatory and safety guidelines for drug safety, pharmaceutical product development, clinical trial design, estimate of product costs, and the perspective on future use of AI in pharmacovigilance.

Keywords: artificial intelligence, pharmacovigilance, data mining, predictive analytics, AI-based evidence generation, data science in pharmacovigilance, machine learning algorithms in pharmacovigilance, natural language processing in pharmacovigilance, pharmacovigilance officer

1. Introduction

Drug-induced morbidity and mortality are among one of the most daunting aspects of pharmacotherapy in daily pharmacy practice; these patients carry the burden of adverse drug reaction (ADR) that ranges from simple urticaria to fatality.

Again, safety of patients has an utmost importance in the practice of day-to-day pharmacotherapy. There should be caution to ensure a balance between risks and benefits of every treatment protocol. Therefore, collaborative efforts should be carried out to detect, evaluate, document, and mitigate adverse drug effects (ADEs). The pharmacovigilance (PV) sciences are focused on the efficacy of drugs and detection of additional adverse events [1, 2].

Pharmacovigilance refers to the practice of monitoring and evaluating medication-induced adverse events. Thus, it works by monitoring and reporting ADEs to the national (local governmental pharmacovigilance centers) [3] as well as international (The Uppsala Monitoring Centre) authorities, thereby identifying it. It is also applied in vaccine safety surveillance. Specifically, the issue of ADR reporting plays a central role in pharmacovigilance. Reporting of ADRs to the regulatory authorities is an important responsibility for healthcare professionals, patients as well as pharmaceutical companies. This information is applied to continuously evaluate medication safety post-marketing [1, 2, 4–6].

Pharmacovigilance is not just about monitoring the benefits and risks of medications throughout their lifecycle. It is about staying ahead of emerging risks. This is where post-marketing surveillance identifies any previously unrecognized adverse effects that may arise when a drug is used in larger populations and for extended periods. Moreover, it is not just about using new technologies such as data mining and artificial intelligence (AI) in pharmacovigilance. It is about how these tools are increasingly used to analyze large amounts of data and detect potential safety signals more efficiently. These advancements help researchers and regulators take appropriate actions to protect public health [4, 5, 7–9].

Early recognition of ADRs by recording and analyzing them systematically may facilitate health professionals in recognizing potential drug safety issues and signal detection to make an appropriate intervention to prevent the occurrence of adverse effects. This proactive stance aims to reduce patient harm and drive overall treatment outcome [3, 7].

Pharmacovigilance is a key to underpin evidence-based care in clinical practice. Ensuring healthcare providers have the most accurate information on the safety and effectiveness of medicines is essential in helping to preserve that confidence in their decision making with respect to prescribing, dispensing, or administering medications to patients. These data help to improve the success of treatments and reduce medication-associated risks [5–8].

Pharmacovigilance, in that sense, quantifies drug-related harm and benefits versus risks to protect the general population from drug-related adverse events. We owe it to those that need evidence-based healthcare, because this joint effort not only ensures the trust from the public in our healthcare systems but also promotes a patient safety culture (accountability in health industry).

Even in the case of pharmacovigilance, data science has become an indispensable element. The vast amounts of data generated in clinical trials, patient records, and post-marketing surveillance can be overwhelming. Data science, by virtue of the sophisticated analytical techniques and computational technologies on which it relies, may facilitate a more efficient approach to processing, analyzing, and interpreting that information in both sectors; extending the reach and effectiveness of regulatory authorities (who have statutory obligations to ensure that pharmaceuticals are safe) as well as from perspective of pharmaceutical companies to improve decision-making capabilities in relation to drug safety [10–12].

The analysis of ADRs is one of the main applications of data science in pharmacovigilance. Traditional methods involved extensive methods of manual reporting and analysis that might be time intensive and miscalculated. This system uses data science, machine learning algorithms, natural language processing (NLP) searching through enormous datasets such as electronic health records (EHRs), and social media posts to recognize potential ADRs earlier in time and more accurately. This automated data extraction and analysis might result in a significantly shorter lead time for identifying, monitoring, and reacting to safety signals.

The comparison of ADR reports from different patients (using artificial intelligence) results in easier utilization of patient-specific risk data, leading to a decrease in the prevalence of ADRs. At the same time, data science techniques and AI tools can be used to integrate into pharmacovigilance systems to enhance the ability for analyzing this abundant patient data and ADR reports, thereby ensuring that high-quality ADR data are collected [10–12].

The reports of adverse drug reactions can be analyzed regularly by AI from a variety of sources such as social media, clinical studies, and electronic health records. AI can identify such patterns and safety signals earlier than traditional methods, and thus aid in faster updating of safety information and in risk minimization associated with medication [11, 13].

In addition to replicating different ADR reporting mechanisms from various countries, an AI-based pharmacovigilance will provide a direction to streamline the global protocol of pharmacovigilance practice. The global focus on these problems emphasizes the need for AI tools and systems to proactively identify both symptom detection algorithms, such as machine learning systems designed to forecast adverse drug events at a population level [14–17].

Through this perspective chapter, we aim to give knowledge and prepare healthcare professionals on how best they can manage such a scenario with the onset of AI-related pharmacovigilance by summarizing the latest literature published from 2015 until now on AI application in pharmacovigilance. We conducted a thorough literature review and selected articles that allowed us to apply the Critical Appraisal Skills Programme (CASP) for critically appraising the literature, rendering secondary data collection and offering new viewpoints on AI in PV following information retrieval [1, 2, 4].

2. Area of application and benefits of AI in pharmacovigilance

2.1 Detection of safety issues and emerging patterns of adverse effects

Adverse medication events (AMEs) or adverse drug reactions (ADRs) are defined as harmful experiences that a patient may undergo following exposure to a medication. They are caused by medication errors, adverse drug reactions, allergic reactions, or overdoses [5–7].

AME signals could be specific indicators for a drug that can cause ADEs in some patients. In the pharmacovigilance field, they are fundamental signals used to detect, analyze, and prevent risks linked with drugs. Sources detecting AME signals include reports from healthcare providers, patient reports, clinical trials, electronic health records (EHRs), literature and studies, and spontaneous reporting system [5, 8, 9]. Once a signal is detected, it undergoes further evaluation to determine causality, frequency, and severity. This may involve statistical analysis, expert review, and additional research. If a significant risk is confirmed, regulatory agencies may take actions such as updating labeling, issuing warnings, or even withdrawing the medication from the market. Identifying AME signals aims to improve patient safety by mitigating risks associated with medication use [3, 8, 9].

Spontaneous reporting systems are a key tool for the identification of AMEs, and this involves healthcare professionals including patients and caregivers. They brought any suspected adverse event to the attention of regulatory bodies, including the U.S. Food and Drug Administration (FDA) MedWatch program or VigiBase of the World Health Organization. These reports provide invaluable real-world data on the safety profile of medications post-marketing. In addition, pharmaceutical companies are bound to perform stumbling pharmacovigilance on their newly developed medications. These data, which is the result of their hard work and dedication, is then collated and analyzed to help identify possible safety signals that could signal wider public health risks [3, 10].

We can exploit those machine learning algorithms, natural language processing (NLP) techniques by incorporating AI models in pharmacovigilance. These systems comprehend vast quantities of unstructured data from sources such as clinical trial reports, medical literature, spontaneous reporting databases, and social media. They can discover patterns, connections, and potential triggers of ADRs at a much faster rate with a higher degree of accuracy than conventional manual modes. AI can, for example, more rapidly flag signals that need follow-up assessment to speed up the regulatory and pharma company response in managing risks with consequences on patient safety [3, 8, 9]. AI has incredible potential to greatly enhance patient safety by detecting subtle patterns and correlations across data that might be missed by a human analysis and can potentially identify adverse events earlier.

DeBERTa, short for Decoding-enhanced BERT with disentangled attention, is a state-of-the-art neural network architecture designed for NLP tasks. This machine learning model aims to quickly and efficiently process large-scale unstructured textual data coming from various sources including medical literature, social media, or adverse events reports. As a result, it can detect drug-associated risks and side effects much faster and more accurately. The self-attentive layers can disentangle different context dependencies, which will benefit in extracting the most closely relative information and relations, and thus lead to an improved means to early detect ADRs [11, 12], offering more favorable risk management and ensuring patient safety. We have explored many NLP algorithms. LSTM and CRF methods were, among these algorithms, the most promising model for detecting adverse medication events [13]. Methods such as NLP allow you to extract useful information from unstructured text data. Consequently, the prediction of ADR risk and severity utilizing predictive modeling functions may enable proactive risk management to ensure patient safety [14, 15]. **Figure 1** explains the process of using ML and NLP for ADR signal detection.

With the help of AI, prescribed medications can be cross-referenced with patient histories and highlight possible allergies, interactions, or contraindications that may result in adverse drug events (ADEs). Utilizing its predictive analytics, a smart, AI platform can determine those patients at highest risk for medication-related harms and thereby enable healthcare professionals to intervene where they can best reduce patient risks. Real-time decision support systems (DSS) can be made to operate based on artificial intelligence, providing such services in real time with evidence-based recommendations and reminders or enforcing compliance with clinical guidelines. AI could help, for example, to recommend better dosing adjustments per renal function of a patient; reduce the risk of overprescribing opioids by having it integrated with

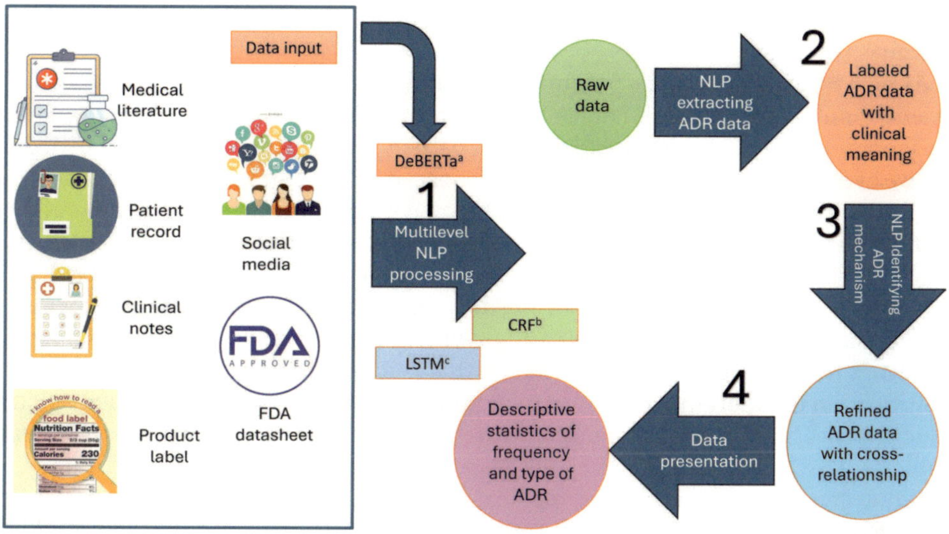

Figure 1.
ADR signal detection and identification of emerging drug safety using machine learning (ML) and natural language processing (NLP): decoding—enhanced BERT with disentangled attention (a), conditional random field (b), and long short-term memory (c).

current clinical data; or even point out situations where alternative therapies are more effective or safer [16, 17].

2.2 Identifying drug-related harm and communicating drug risks using AI

Using sophisticated algorithms such as neural networks, decision trees, clustering techniques, each regulatory body and pharma company can unearth more patterns and correlations that traditional methods may overlook. With such systems, we can quickly respond to new data, and potentially set up for real-time surveillance or interventions. Anomaly detection models, for instance, can be employed to flag unanticipated spikes in the frequency of ADRs, which require further scrutiny. In conclusion, machine learning improves the general efficiency of pharmacovigilance systems guaranteeing that efficient and safe therapeutics are available for patients at the same time reducing the danger of negative health outcomes [14, 15].

AI-powered predictive analytics for drug safety in pharmaceutical is an emerging and innovative concept. Powered by sophisticated machine learning, such analytics are capable of quickly and accurately analyzing large amounts of data. By taking this proactive, data-driven approach, pharmaceutical companies and regulatory agencies can better predict drug reactions sooner, which can improve patient safety and allow more informed decisions to be made over the course of new potential drug development processes [18, 19]. With the aid of predictive analytics, it helps in the real-time monitoring of drug safety and automatically detects any emerging safety issues. Predictive analytics uses advanced algorithms and machine learning methods to identify the signals of abnormality that would not have been recognized through conventional surveillance approaches [19, 20]. They will greatly increase the efficiency and effectiveness of safety surveillance efforts. Direct insights from heterogeneous data enable real-time detection of signals and events related to the safety. The early discovery of this association can also prompt regulatory action and risk management strategies hence ultimately lessening harm to patients and improving public health outcomes [18, 21].

AI may transform how the potential risks of drugs are communicated in specific patient populations. Its reach is such that it can combine details of socio-demographics, genome profiles, medical histories, and patient prescriptions to give a 360-degree picture of how well a population is. The purpose of this integration is to facilitate the identification of potential sub-populations in which health-related events might occur more frequently for given patients characteristics. This level of detailed analysis is important for identifying risk factors that would otherwise not be detected, such as rarer genetic variants or multiple drug interactions in a patient. AI systems can refresh their predictive models to align with these new real-world data and any new drugs that were introduced. However, this dynamic adaptation enables timely identification of emerging drug safety signals, which in turn supports proactive harm reduction measures to be put in place before issues escalate to the level of widespread problems. Further, AI can predict drug responses based on patient-specific data including genetic information and medical history. As a result, AI models can detect patients with increased risk of adverse reactions to specific drugs and offer individual warnings or recommendations for drug substitutions [16, 17, 22–24].

The AI tools and systems to quantify drug-related patient harm are outlined in **Table 1**.

Patient-centered drug risk communication could be a major stomping ground for AI. This is done by using AI systems and tools to assess patient data for risk factors (medication allergies), so that this balance of risks versus benefits can be assessed

AI/machine learning system	Description	Use	Reference
aTarantula	NLP tool using context-based machine learning algorithm to extract ADR data from social media	Detection of safety issues and emerging patterns of adverse effects	[25]
TF-IDF	NLP algorithm to detect ADR		[22]
LGBM	ML algorithm to detect ADR		[17]
XLM	Self-supervised ML model to detect ADR		[8]
FastText	Unsupervised ML model to identify ADR seriousness of ADR		[26]
CamemBERT	ML model to identify ADR seriousness of ADR		[25]
BERT	NLP model to classify ADR		[27]
GPT	NLP model to classify ADR		[28]
BioBERT	NLP model to classify ADR		[29]
XLNet	NLP model to classify ADR		[30, 31]
BERT	NLP model to classify ADR	Identifying drug-related harm and communicating drug risks	[31]
GPT	NLP model to classify ADR		[32]
NER	NLP identify and classify entities in text, such as drug names, patient symptoms, and adverse reactions		[33]

AI/machine learning system	Description	Use	Reference
RF	ML model to generate ICSR reports automatically	Used in regulatory decision making in drug safety	[34]
SVM	ML model to generate ICSR reports automatically		[24]
GBM	ML model to generate ICSR reports automatically		[29]
Neural network	ML model to generate ICSR reports automatically		[35]
			[23]
RNNs	Deep learning model to predict ADR	AI model used in active surveillance of drug safety issues	[36]
CNNs	Deep learning model to predict ADR		[37]
Autoencoders	Deep learning model to predict ADR		[21]
Time-Series Analysis	Detecting changes in trends that may signal a safety issue.		[37]
ClinicalBERT	NLP extracting and analyzing clinical trial texts and medical literature	Clinical trial design	[38]
Survival Analysis Models Cox Proportional Hazards Model	NLP and ML model for time-to-event data analyses in clinical trail		[39]
DNNs	Applied broadly for predicting molecular properties and disease outcomes from large datasets	New drug screening and pharmaceutical product development	[1]
DeepChem	An open-source toolkit that uses deep learning for drug discovery, materials science, and quantum chemistry		[40]
AlphaFold	Predicts protein structures with high accuracy, which is crucial for understanding biological functions and drug interactions		[28]

BERT (Bidirectional Encoder Representations from Transformers), GPT (Generative Pre-trained Transformer), NER (Named Entity Recognition), TF-IDF (Term Frequency-Inverse Document Frequency), XLM Cross-lingual Language, LGBM (Light Gradient Boosted Machine), NLP (natural language processing), NER (Named Entity Recognition), RF (Random Forests), SVM (Support Vector Machines), GBM (Gradient Boosting Machines), DNNs (Deep Neural Networks).

Table 1.
List of AI tools and systems used in pharmacovigilance practices.

on an individual patient basis. As such, they do not serve to provide clinicians with definitive answers on patient therapies [17, 22].

2.3 Regulatory decision making in drug safety using AI

Pharmacovigilance, an important area of drug safety, is one such field that benefits significantly from artificial intelligence, a major player in regulatory decision-making and drug regulatory authorities. AI offers Regulatory Intelligence, utilizing NLP and machine learning systems for detecting regulatory changes. In addition to the capability of extracting information from free text, AI can fill in the knowledge gaps of drug safety and regulations on a global level for pharmaceutical companies allowing building successful strategies [23, 34].

AI can also simplify reporting of adverse events and automatically generate/ adapt reports for submission in a standardized and consistent manner, hence reducing workload from healthcare professionals and resulting on higher data collection efficiency. The use of AI tools can help regulatory authorities review safety data from drug companies at a faster and more accurate pace to identify emerging risks that require mitigation [5, 13].

Post-Market Continuous AI-driven Monitoring: Real-time surveillance post-market can detect early signals of adverse events and respond timely to protect public health. In addition, AI can assist with the triage of safety signals for prioritization of signal evaluation due to its relative potential impact and likelihood, respectively enhancing the signal detection capacity for sponsors highlighting critical issues [8, 12].

The effects of AI are broader, and one example is personalized patient care where it helps in identifying individuals who are at risk forms for specific reactions. AI also improves care quality by recommending individualized interventions or providers to monitor [6]. Furthermore, AI tools give a helping hand to pharmaceutical companies in abidance of the legal norms by automatizing the report generation and making sure that material is submitted into relevant regulatory bodies on time [23].

This AI-led revolution helps in aiding the drug discovery process thereby recognizing high safety profile of drug development candidates. In turn, this approach allows sponsors to proactively monitor AEs throughout clinical trial execution once a product is on the market. AI also contributes to decision-making tools for regulatory agencies and pharmaceutical companies, delivering evidence-based decisions on drug safety by improving the aggregation and mining of data [10, 17].

Pharmacovigilance regulatory compliance requires detailed and accurate documentation as well as submission of reports to various regulatory bodies. A significant component of it can be automated with AI, so the reports are accurate, consistent, and timely. With automated report generation systems, data can be aggregated, relevant analysis executed, and the results formatted as required by regulatory standards from various countries. This automation alleviates compliance burdens on pharma companies, reduces attempts for human error, and guarantees regulators the data they need to make informed decisions about drug safety.

The generation of Individual Case Safety Reports (ICSRs) involves the precise extraction of relevant data from various sources, such as EHRs and patient reports. AI technologies, specifically natural language processing (NLP), play an instrumental role in automating this process. NLP algorithms can parse through unstructured text, identifying and extracting crucial information. This automation increases efficiency and ensures that no critical data are overlooked, providing a comprehensive foundation for ICSR generation [14, 33]. Automated generation of ICSRs reports and reporting drug-related safety issues using AI models are described in **Figure 2**.

2.4 AI-based pharmacovigilance activities in drug therapy

The field of artificial intelligence (AI) has the potential to uncover variations in how patients respond to drug treatments. This is achieved through the use of advanced AI algorithms and machine learning methods that can process and analyze large volumes of biological, genetic, and clinical data. These algorithms identify patterns that are not detectable through conventional methods. This enables a more

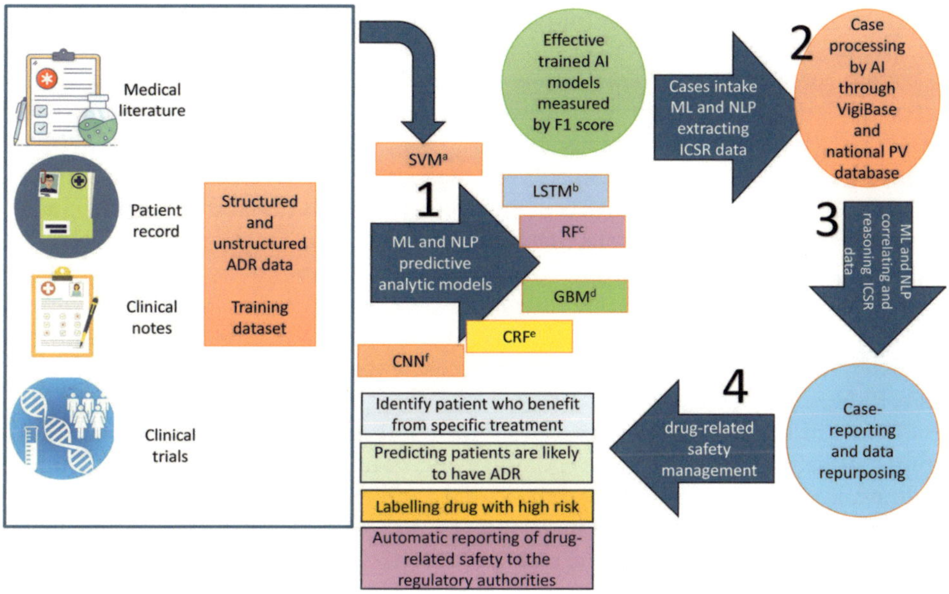

Figure 2.
Generating individual case safety reports (ICSRs) and drug-related safety management using artificial intelligence (AI): support vector machines (a), long short-term memory (b), random forest (c), gradient boosting machines (d), conditional random fields (e), and convolutional neural networks (f).

nuanced understanding of why different patients respond differently to the same medication, paving the way for more personalized and effective treatments [1, 2, 4].

AI is a potent use case to predict patient response for specific drugs when coupled with genomics sciences. Such methods of deep learning can consider thousands of genetic markers simultaneously and connect them with drug response data to identify specific genetic signatures associated with efficacy or toxicity [1, 2, 4]. This real-world implementation of AI based on individual patient data for drug response prediction is an important breakthrough in personalized medicine.

By mining electronic health records, AI can identify how patients respond to treatments over time while accounting for variables such as age, sex, comorbid conditions, and concomitant medications. This will guide machine learning algorithms to predict which patients are going to respond best to which drugs and optimize therapeutic strategies. This use of real-world data can identify less common but important trends that may be underpowered by controlled clinical trials, lending additional depth and iteration to the results [1, 2].

AI can mimic responses of diverse human cell types and genetic backgrounds to candidate drugs, forecasting distinct population-specific effects and providing information on the biological and environmental variables that may be driving drug response. This will be very important for the development of real personalized medicine, where therapies are made considering the peculiarities of each patient [1, 4].

2.5 Application of AI in active surveillance of safety issues

Timely monitoring and signal detection are two significant advantages of AI in pharmacovigilance for the real-time surveillance of adverse drug reactions. Artificial intelligence (AI) is one of the advanced technologies that could be incorporated in clinical decision support tools to notify healthcare providers about possible ADRs while prescribing. For example, AI can identify that a newly prescribed drug has high interaction risk with the patient's foundation medications and doctor can change treatment plan before it becomes intuitive to use or find out that the patient does not respond positively due to an already existing medications. This kind of life-saving evidence-based alert can significantly reduce the risk associated with ADRs. There is continuous monitoring of the EHRs using predictive analytics and natural language processing (NLP) to spot patterns that reflect in poor drug reactions. Examples include NLP for interpreting physicians' notes and patients' comments to identify ADRs at an early stage that are not detected by traditional methods [41–44].

In this digital age, with all the scientific advancements that are happening around us and driven by cutting-edge research in data sciences, several regulatory agencies (FDA, EMA) have started using AI-powered techniques for real-time post-market surveillance of their drug safety profiles. The use of AI is crucial for promptly identifying new safety signals so that regulatory decisions (e.g., label changes or drug withdrawals) are based on the most up-to-date and extensive dataset possible. It will be essential, as a previous study illustrated [41, 42], that such AI-driven continuous monitoring occurs to ensure public trust in pharmaceutical interventions.

The strengthening of post-marketing surveillance helps to detect ADRs occurring after the release of a drug into the market, thereby increasing the participation and usefulness of AI. The scale and scope of surveillance enabled by AI are obviously far beyond the reach of individuals to carry out with their own efforts in collecting and analyzing large aspects of data within widespread and heterogeneous populations. DL uses machine learning models (the tool behind AI) to make predictions about the likelihood of an ADR based on historical data and trends, information that could ultimately guide regulatory decision making as well as influence medical practice. Together with AI, this big data approach allows the understanding of how diverse populations from around the world may experience a medication in their everyday life [41–44].

By analyzing patient-specific factors, AI helps in the integration of personalized medicine into active surveillance systems for ADRs. This personalized analysis further aids in predicting who is more likely to develop certain ADRs and affect the prescription of drug use. The identification of these personalized risk factors allows healthcare providers to use them as the basis for more informed decisions, increasing patient safety and treatment efficacy [41, 42].

2.6 Clinical trial design using AI

Advanced artificial intelligence (AI) algorithms along with advanced machine learning techniques can process thousands of data records, identify complex patterns, and derive the future predictions more accurately. These abilities turn to designing more efficient trials, being able to allocate resources in an optimal way as well as all in all improving the general reliability of the results. AI-powered analytics can assist patient recruitment and selection by using EHR, genetic data, and other information to quickly detect the most appropriate candidates. Since machine learning models can forecast patient eligibility *via* inclusion and exclusion criteria, this aligns well with a more focused recruitment strategy [38, 39].

It is through AI that different scenario for a trial can be envisaged and then optimized by predicting future potentially outcomes along with their probabilities. Advanced algorithms analyze historical trial data, real-world evidence, and current scientific literature to propose optimal trial designs ensuring efficacy, safety, and cost. By selecting studies that are not too underpowered or whose patient response is very scattered, AI systems can help ensure the probability of conclusive and reproducible results [38, 39, 45].

AI can be integrated for clinical trial Design: AI-driven outcomes analysis could help to improve the results of a clinical trial. Specifically, AI models can predict the outcomes and safety of new treatments before the trial concludes. This is important as these predictions assist researchers in determining whether to continue, modify, or terminate a trial. It can also be used to learn subpopulations of patients who respond differently to treatment on complex datasets (AI in medicine) and enable personalized medicine paradigms [38, 45].

2.7 New drug screening and pharmaceutical product development using AI

AI-driven approaches are revolutionizing drug discovery and development, offering unprecedented speed and efficiency. By simulating the interactions of potential drugs with various human cell types and genetic backgrounds, AI can predict diverse responses across different populations. Through virtual screening and *in silico* trials, AI swiftly and effectively identifies promising compounds, expediting the pipeline from discovery to clinical use [40, 46].

AI harnesses the power of machine learning algorithms to accurately predict the biological activity of compounds. By scrutinizing patterns and relationships within extensive datasets, AI can swiftly identify promising drug candidates, surpassing the capabilities of conventional methods. Moreover, AI-driven models enhance the precision of drug screening by accurately predicting the binding affinity of drug molecules to their target proteins. Techniques such as deep learning and neural networks, trained on existing datasets of known drug-target interactions, can predict how new compounds will interact with specific biological targets [40, 46, 47].

One of the most significant impacts of AI in new drug screening is its potential to facilitate the discovery of novel drug candidates through generative modeling. AI can be harnessed to design new molecules with desired pharmacological properties from the ground up, leveraging techniques such as reinforcement learning and generative adversarial networks (GANs). These AI-generated compounds can then be evaluated for their potential efficacy and safety, opening up a new frontier for drug discovery that transcends the modification of existing molecules [13, 40, 46, 47].

AI can also provide insights into the mechanistic basis of adverse drug reactions. By integrating various data types, including genomic, proteomic, and metabolic data, AI systems can uncover underlying biological mechanisms that predispose patients to specific ADRs. For example, AI can identify genetic variants contributing to drug hypersensitivity or metabolic pathways resulting in toxic metabolites. Machine learning models can predict these associations by learning from large-scale datasets, generating hypotheses for further experimental validation. This understanding allows for the development of more precise and personalized drug therapy that can avoid adverse reactions and reduce toxicity. AI's ability to identify patterns in complex and high-dimensional data can provide insights into the molecular and cellular pathways involved in ADRs, thus enhancing our understanding of drug safety and paving the way for more effective interventions [13, 46–48].

Connectomic analysis, which maps the connections in the brain, can be enhanced with AI to understand how certain drugs impact neural circuits at a cellular level, potentially leading to ADRs. For example, neurotoxicity is a common ADR for many therapeutic agents. By analyzing large-scale neural network data, AI can help identify specific neural pathways disrupted by drug interactions, informing safer drug design and targeted therapies. This capability is compelling in psychopharmacology, where the intricate interplay between neurotransmitter systems and drug targets often presents a high risk of adverse effects [13, 46].

AI algorithms can analyze proteomic and metabolomic profiles to identify biomarkers that predict adverse drug reactions. These biomarkers can provide early warnings during clinical trials or clinical settings, allowing for timely interventions. By understanding the changes in protein and metabolic levels, researchers can also gain valuable insights into the mechanisms driving ADRs, contributing to the development of safer drugs [46–48].

AI-driven drug repurposing efforts can benefit from an enhanced understanding of ADR mechanisms. Using AI to analyze adverse reactions, researchers can predict potential ADRs for existing drugs tested for new therapeutic purposes. Identifying such risks early can prevent similar outcomes in new therapeutic contexts. Moreover, understanding the mechanistic basis of ADRs can reveal off-target effects central to the repurposing strategy, ensuring a more comprehensive safety profile for the repurposed drugs [47, 48]. Improving exiting drug safety, screening new drug, and enhancing personalized drug therapy are described in **Figure 3**.

2.8 List of AI tools and systems used in pharmacovigilance

Based on the argument detailed in the present perspective chapter, integrating AI into pharmacovigilance is highly important for healthcare providers, pharmacovigilance experts, and regulatory authorities. Given the importance of drug safety

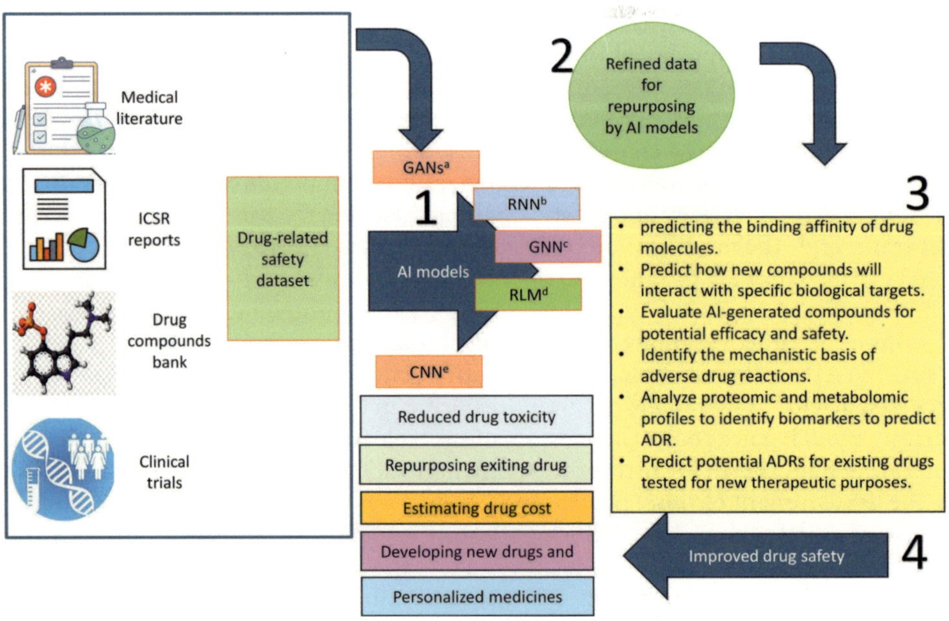

Figure 3.
Improving safety of exiting drugs and screening of new drugs using AI models: generative adversarial networks (a), recurrent neural networks (b), graph neural networks (c), reinforcement learning models (d), and convolutional neural networks (e).

to the public and the accelerating progression of developing AI-related sciences, it would be essential to list the most significant AI models and systems used in pharmacovigilance. **Table 1** lists the AI tools and systems used to improve the capabilities of pharmacovigilance practices.

3. Challenges and barriers of integrating artificial intelligence into pharmacovigilance

Integrating artificial intelligence (AI) into pharmacovigilance poses several significant challenges and barriers that need to be addressed to fully realize its potential. Firstly, data quality and consistency present a major hurdle. These datasets are often heterogeneous, incomplete, and unstructured, making it difficult for AI systems to extract meaningful insights. Ensuring that data are clean, accurate, and harmonized is crucial but resource-intensive, requiring substantial investments in data preprocessing and standardization. Another significant challenge is the need for transparency and interpretability in AI algorithms. Regulatory bodies such as the FDA and EMA place a high emphasis on the explainability of safety assessment processes. AI models, particularly complex ones like deep learning networks, often operate as "black boxes," making it challenging to understand how they derive their conclusions [24, 28, 45].

Regulatory and ethical considerations also pose significant challenges. The use of AI in pharmacovigilance involves processing sensitive health data, raising concerns about patient privacy and data security. Ensuring compliance with regulations such as the GDPR in Europe and HIPAA in the United States is essential to protect patient confidentiality. Moreover, ethical considerations regarding the deployment of AI in healthcare must be addressed, such as ensuring unbiased algorithms that do not perpetuate existing health disparities. Developing ethical guidelines and standards for the use of AI in pharmacovigilance is imperative to address these concerns [24, 45, 49].

Technical limitations in AI technology itself act as barriers. For instance, current natural language processing (NLP) algorithms, which are essential for analyzing unstructured text data like medical reports, still struggle with the complexity and variability of medical language. These algorithms need to be continuously refined to accurately capture the nuances of medical terminology and context. Additionally, integrating AI with existing pharmacovigilance software and IT infrastructure can be challenging, requiring significant technical expertise and investment. Overcoming these technical barriers is crucial for the seamless incorporation of AI into pharmacovigilance systems [24, 49, 50].

Moreover, technical challenges in training datasets and validation of artificial intelligence for pharmacovigilance were implied. Robust validation of AI models in pharmacovigilance is essential to ensure their reliability and generalizability. Standard validation methods, such as cross-validation and bootstrapping, may not fully capture the complexity of real-world scenarios. It is necessary to use a combination of internal validation (using part of the training data) and external validation (using independent datasets) to comprehensively assess model performance. Standardizing terminologies using medical dictionaries (like MedDRA or SNOMED CT) and developing sophisticated data normalization techniques are essential steps to overcome this challenge. A majority of the available data pertains to normal, non-adverse outcomes, while only a small fraction relates to ADRs. Training AI models on such imbalanced datasets can result in poor performance, as the models may become biased toward the majority class and fail to detect ADRs accurately. Text in medical records often includes domain-specific jargon, abbreviations, and complex sentence structures, posing significant challenges for standard NLP techniques. Advances in NLP, such as transformer-based models and contextual embeddings, offer promising solutions, but their application to specialized domains like pharmacovigilance requires careful tuning and validation [24, 28, 45, 49, 50].

4. Future perspectives

AI models and systems have implied a significant contribution in improving drug-related safety through integration with pharmacovigilance. However, to enhance the performance of AI applications in pharmacovigilance, expert should consider these strategies:

1. Quality data: Utilize high-quality, diverse datasets to train AI models effectively. Incorporate structured and unstructured data sources for a comprehensive understanding.

2. Continuous learning: Implement models that can adapt and learn from new data. Techniques such as transfer learning and reinforcement learning can enhance AI's ability to recognize patterns and trends.

3. Interpretability: Aim for models that provide explanations for their predictions. This transparency is vital in pharmacovigilance to understand how decisions are made.

4. Collaboration: Foster collaboration between AI experts, pharmacovigilance specialists, and domain experts to leverage diverse perspectives. This interdisciplinary approach can lead to more robust AI solutions.

5. Regulatory compliance: Ensure AI applications meet regulatory requirements and standards in the healthcare industry. Compliance with data privacy laws like GDPR is crucial.

6. Feedback loops: Establish mechanisms to receive feedback from end users on AI predictions. These data can be used to fine-tune models and improve accuracy over time.

5. Conclusions

Incorporating artificial intelligence (AI) into pharmacovigilance practices represents a major advancement in improving drug safety and public health. Pharmacovigilance, which involves the continuous monitoring, assessment, and prevention of adverse effects associated with pharmaceutical products, stands to gain tremendously from AI's powerful capabilities in data processing and pattern recognition. AI algorithms have the ability to efficiently analyze immense volumes of data originating from diverse sources, including various types of clinical studies, medical records, and social media, with unprecedented speed and accuracy. This capability allows for the early identification of potential adverse drug reactions (ADRs), providing a proactive approach to drug safety monitoring. By automating routine tasks, AI not only reduces the time and cost associated with pharmacovigilance but also enables human experts to focus on more complex analyses, thereby increasing the overall efficiency and effectiveness of the pharmacovigilance system.

Moreover, AI's capacity for continuous learning and improvement further underscores its value in pharmacovigilance. Advanced machine learning models can adapt over time, improving their predictive accuracy as new data become available. This dynamic capability is crucial in the constantly evolving landscape of drug safety, where new ADRs can emerge as drugs are used by larger and more diverse populations. Additionally, AI-driven systems can facilitate better regulatory compliance by providing comprehensive and timely reports required by health authorities. They can also enhance signal detection processes, aiding in the rapid identification of safety concerns that might be missed by traditional methods. As the pharmaceutical industry continues to grapple with the complexities of monitoring drug safety, the integration of AI into pharmacovigilance not only promises to safeguard patient health more effectively but also to revolutionize the way drug safety data is handled and interpreted.

Here are some key aspects of applying AI in pharmacovigilance:

1. Early detection of ADRs: AI algorithms have the capability to process and examine massive amounts of data gathered from diverse sources such as social media, electronic health records, and medical literature. This allows them to detect potential adverse drug reactions (ADRs) at an early stage, enabling prompt intervention when necessary.

2. Signal detection: AI tools can help in signal detection by analyzing patterns in data to identify potential safety concerns related to specific drugs or medical products.

3. Risk assessment: AI can assist in risk assessment by predicting which patients may be at a higher risk of experiencing certain ADRs, allowing for personalized monitoring and prevention strategies.

4. Automation of reporting: AI can automate the collection, processing, and reporting of ADR data, improving the efficiency and accuracy of pharmacovigilance activities.

5. Data mining and analysis: AI techniques such as natural language processing (NLP) can extract valuable insights from unstructured data such as patient reports, medical records, and scientific literature, enhancing pharmacovigilance surveillance.

6. Enhanced pharmacovigilance surveillance: AI systems can continuously monitor large datasets for safety signals, enabling real-time pharmacovigilance surveillance and rapid response to emerging safety issues.

Overall, the application of AI in pharmacovigilance can lead to more proactive and effective monitoring of drug safety, ultimately improving patient outcomes and regulatory decision making.

Currently, there are challenges and limitations in fully integrating AI models and systems into pharmacovigilance. These include issues with data quality, as data sources may be varied and contain errors, missing information, or inconsistencies. These issues can impact the performance of AI algorithms. Additionally, AI algorithms have the potential to perpetuate biases present in the data they are trained on. In pharmacovigilance, biased data can lead to skewed results and inaccurate predictions, potentially affecting patient safety, and the use of AI in pharmacovigilance raises regulatory challenges, as agencies need to establish standards for validating AI algorithms and ensuring patient safety. Current regulations may not be adequately equipped to address the unique characteristics of AI technologies.

Conflict of interest

The authors declare no conflict of interest.

Author details

Mohamed Gamaleldin[1*], Shaimaa Abdelhalim[1] and Ivo Abraham[2,3,4,5]

1 Department of Pharmaceutical Sciences (Pharm-D Program), Fakeeh College for Medical Sciences, Jeddah, Saudi Arabia

2 Department of Pharmacy Practice and Science, R. K. Coit College of Pharmacy, University of Arizona, Tucson, Arizona, USA

3 Department of Family and Community Medicine, College of Medicine, University of Arizona, Tucson, Arizona, USA

4 Clinical Translational Sciences, University of Arizona Health Sciences, Arizona, USA

5 Matrix45, Tucson, AZ, USA

*Address all correspondence to: mgamaleldin@fcms.edu.sa

IntechOpen

© 2024 The Author(s). Licensee IntechOpen. This chapter is distributed under the terms of the Creative Commons Attribution License (http://creativecommons.org/licenses/by/4.0), which permits unrestricted use, distribution, and reproduction in any medium, provided the original work is properly cited.

References

[1] Singh S, Kumar R, Payra S, Singh SK. Artificial intelligence and machine learning in pharmacological research: Bridging the gap between data and drug discovery. Cureus [Internet]. 2023;**15**(8):e44359. Available from: https://pubmed.ncbi.nlm.nih.gov/37779744/ [Accessed: June 21, 2024]

[2] Ahmad T, Lund LH, Rao P, Ghosh R, Warier P, Vaccaro B, et al. Machine learning methods improve prognostication, identify clinically distinct phenotypes, and detect heterogeneity in response to therapy in a large cohort of heart failure patients. Journal of the American Heart Association [Internet]. 2018;**7**(8). Available from: https://www.ahajournals.org/doi/abs/10.1161/JAHA.117.008081 [Accessed: June 21, 2024]

[3] Zhan C, Roughead E, Liu L, Pratt N, Li J. Detecting potential signals of adverse drug events from prescription data. Artificial Intelligence in Medicine [Internet]. 2020;**104**. Available from: https://pubmed.ncbi.nlm.nih.gov/32499007/ [Accessed: June 3, 2024]

[4] Senthil Kumar K, Miskovic V, Blasiak A, Sundar R, Pedrocchi ALG, Pearson AT, et al. Artificial intelligence in clinical oncology: From data to digital pathology and treatment. American Society of Clinical Oncology Educational [Internet]. 2023;**43**:e390084. Available from: https://ascopubs.org/doi/10.1200/EDBK_390084 [Accessed: June 21, 2024]

[5] Skelly CL, Cassagnol M, Munakomi S. Adverse Events [Internet]. Treasure Island (FL): StatPearls Publishing; 2023. pp. 213-221. Available from: https://www.ncbi.nlm.nih.gov/books/NBK558963/ [Accessed: June 21, 2024]

[6] Laatikainen O, Sneck S, Turpeinen M. Medication-related adverse events in health care—What have we learned? A narrative overview of the current knowledge. European Journal of Clinical Pharmacology [Internet]. 2022;**78**(2):159. Available from: https://pmc/articles/PMC8748358/ [Accessed: June 3, 2024]

[7] Montané E, Santesmases J. Adverse drug reactions. Medicina Clínica (Barc) [Internet]. 2020;**154**(5):178-184. Available from: https://pubmed.ncbi.nlm.nih.gov/31771857/ [Accessed: June 3, 2024]

[8] Hoang T, Liu J, Roughead E, Pratt N, Li J. Supervised signal detection for adverse drug reactions in medication dispensing data. Computer Methods and Programs in Biomedicine [Internet]. 2018;**161**:25-38. Available from: https://pubmed.ncbi.nlm.nih.gov/29852965/ Accessed: June 3, 2024

[9] Loke YK, Mattishent K, Navaneetharaja N. New adverse drug reaction signals from 2017 to 2021—Genuine alerts or false alarms? Pharmacy [Internet]. 2024;**12**(1):33. Available from: https://pmc/articles/PMC10892108/ [Accessed: June 3, 2024]

[10] Sartori D, Aronson JK, Onakpoya IJ. Signals of adverse drug reactions communicated by pharmacovigilance stakeholders: Protocol for a scoping review of the global literature. Systematic Reviews [Internet]. 2020;**9**(1). Available from: https://pmc/articles/PMC7425142/ [Accessed: June 3, 2024]

[11] McMaster C, Chan J, Liew DFL, Su E, Frauman AG, Chapman WW, et al. Developing a deep learning natural language processing algorithm for automated reporting of adverse

drug reactions. Journal of Biomedical Informatics [Internet]. 2023:137. Available from: https://pubmed.ncbi.nlm.nih.gov/36464227/ [Accessed: June 3, 2024]

[12] Pilipiec P, Liwicki M, Bota A. Using machine learning for pharmacovigilance: A systematic review. Pharmaceutics [Internet]. 2022;**14**(2). Available from: https://pmc/articles/PMC8924891/ [Accessed: June 3, 2024]

[13] Murphy RM, Klopotowska JE, de Keizer NF, Jager KJ, Leopold JH, Dongelmans DA, et al. Adverse drug event detection using natural language processing: A scoping review of supervised learning methods. PLoS One [Internet]. 2023;**18**(1). Available from: https://pmc/articles/PMC9810201/ [Accessed: June 4, 2024]

[14] Woodman RJ, Mangoni AA. A comprehensive review of machine learning algorithms and their application in geriatric medicine: Present and future. Aging Clinical and Experimental Research [Internet]. 2023;**35**(11):2363. Available from: https://pmc/articles/PMC10627901/ [Accessed: June 4, 2024]

[15] Sarker IH. Machine learning: Algorithms, real-world applications and research directions. SN Computer Science [Internet]. 2021;**2**(3):160. Available from: https://pmc/articles/PMC7983091/ [Accessed: June 4, 2024]

[16] Härkänen M, Haatainen K, Vehviläinen-Julkunen K, Miettinen M. Artificial intelligence for identifying the prevention of medication incidents causing serious or moderate harm: An analysis using incident reporters' views. International Journal of Environmental Research and Public Health [Internet]. 2021;**18**(17). Available from: https://pmc/articles/PMC8431329/ [Accessed: June 20, 2024]

[17] Choudhury A, Asan O. Role of artificial intelligence in patient safety outcomes: Systematic literature review. JMIR Medical Informatics [Internet]. 2020;**8**(7). Available from: https://pmc/articles/PMC7414411/ [Accessed: June 20, 2024]

[18] Liu VX, Bates DW, Wiens J, Shah NH. The number needed to benefit: Estimating the value of predictive analytics in healthcare. Journal of the American Medical Informatics Association [Internet]. 2019;**26**(12):1655. Available from: https://pmc/articles/PMC6857505/ [Accessed: June 4, 2024]

[19] Lamy JB. A data science approach to drug safety: Semantic and visual mining of adverse drug events from clinical trials of pain treatments. Artificial Intelligence in Medicine [Internet]. 2021;**115**. Available from: https://pubmed.ncbi.nlm.nih.gov/34001324/ [Accessed: June 4, 2024]

[20] Smith GF. Artificial intelligence in drug safety and metabolism. Methods in Molecular Biology [Internet]. 2022;**2390**:483-501. Available from: https://pubmed.ncbi.nlm.nih.gov/34731484/ [Accessed: June 4, 2024]

[21] De Abreu FR, Zhong S, Moureaud C, Le MT, Rothstein A, Li X, et al. A pilot, predictive surveillance model in pharmacovigilance using machine learning approaches. Advances in Therapy [Internet]. 2024;**41**(6):2435. Available from: https://pmc/articles/PMC11133112/ [Accessed: June 4, 2024]

[22] Fisher A, Young MM, Payer D, Pacheco K, Dubeau C, Mago V. Automating detection of drug-related harms on social media: Machine learning framework. Journal of Medical Internet Research [Internet]. 2023;**25**(1). Available from: https://pmc/articles/PMC10548323/ [Accessed: June 20, 2024]

[23] Li M, Chen S, Lai Y, Liang Z, Wang J, Shi J, et al. Integrating real-world evidence in the regulatory decision-making process: A systematic analysis of experiences in the US, EU, and China using a logic model. Frontiers in Medicine [Internet]. 2021;**8**:669509. Available from: https://pmc/articles/PMC8200400/ [Accessed: June 20, 2024]

[24] Desai MK. Artificial intelligence in pharmacovigilance – Opportunities and challenges. Perspectives in Clinical Research [Internet]. 2024;**15**(3):116-121. Available from: https://journals.lww.com/picp/fulltext/9900/artificial_intelligence_in_pharmacovigilance__.18.aspx [Accessed: June 15, 2024]

[25] Roosan D, Law AV, Roosan MR, Li Y. Artificial intelligent context-aware machine-learning tool to detect adverse drug events from social media platforms. Journal of Medical Toxicology [Internet]. 2022;**18**(4):311. Available from: https://pmc/articles/PMC9492823/ [Accessed: June 22, 2024]

[26] Ghosh R, Kempf D, Pufko A, Barrios Martinez LF, Davis CM, Sethi S. Automation opportunities in pharmacovigilance: An industry survey. Pharmaceutical Medicine [Internet]. 2020;**34**(1):7-18. Available from: https://pubmed.ncbi.nlm.nih.gov/32036574/ [Accessed: June 21, 2024]

[27] Alsanosi SM, Padmanabhan S. Potential applications of artificial intelligence (AI) in managing polypharmacy in Saudi Arabia: A narrative review. Healthcare [Internet]. 2024;**12**(7). Available from: https://pmc/articles/PMC11011812/ [Accessed: June 22, 2024]

[28] Crisafulli S, Ciccimarra F, Bellitto C, Carollo M, Carrara E, Stagi L, et al. Artificial intelligence for optimizing benefits and minimizing risks of pharmacological therapies: Challenges and opportunities. Frontiers in Drug Safety and Regulation. 2024;**4**:1356405

[29] Kara V, Powell G, Mahaux O, Jayachandra A, Nyako N, Golds C, et al. Finding needles in the haystack: Clinical utility score for prioritisation (CUSP), an automated approach for identifying spontaneous reports with the highest clinical utility. Drug Safety [Internet]. 2023;**46**(9):847. Available from: https://pmc/articles/PMC10442257/ [Accessed: June 22, 2024]

[30] Aronson JK. Artificial intelligence in pharmacovigilance: An introduction to terms, concepts, applications, and limitations. Drug Safety [Internet]. 2022;**45**(5):407-418. Available from: https://pubmed.ncbi.nlm.nih.gov/35579806/ [Accessed: June 3, 2024]

[31] Chalasani SH, Syed J, Ramesh M, Patil V, Pramod Kumar TM. Artificial intelligence in the field of pharmacy practice: A literature review. Exploratory Research in Clinical and Social Pharmacy [Internet]. 2023;**12**. Available from: https://pmc/articles/PMC10598710/ [Accessed: June 4, 2024]

[32] Noguchi Y, Tachi T, Teramachi H. Detection algorithms and attentive points of safety signal using spontaneous reporting systems as a clinical data source. Briefings in Bioinformatics [Internet]. 2021;**22**(6). Available from: https://pubmed.ncbi.nlm.nih.gov/34453158/ [Accessed: June 4, 2024]

[33] Kim HR, Sung M, Park JA, Jeong K, Kim HH, Lee S, et al. Analyzing adverse drug reaction using statistical and machine learning methods: A systematic review. Medicine (Baltimore) [Internet]. 2022;**101**(25):E29387. Available from: https://pmc/articles/PMC9276413/ [Accessed: June 4, 2024]

[34] Ahuja V, Alvarez CA, Birge JR, Syverson C. Enhancing regulatory decision making for postmarket drug safety. Management Science [Internet]. 2021;**67**(12):7493-7510. Available from: https://pubsonline.informs.org/doi/abs/10.1287/mnsc.2020.3889 [Accessed: June 20, 2024]

[35] Lee VC. Big data and pharmacovigilance: Data mining for adverse drug events and interactions. Pharmacology & Therapeutics [Internet]. 2018;**43**(6):340. Available from: https://pmc/articles/PMC5969211/ [Accessed: June 4, 2024]

[36] Iqbal MZ, Faiz MFI. Active surveillance for COVID-19 through artificial intelligence using real-time speech-recognition mobile application. In: 2020 IEEE International Conference on Consumer Electronics - Taiwan, ICCE-Taiwan. IEEE; 2020

[37] Nayan M, Salari K, Bozzo A, Ganglberger W, Lu G, Carvalho F, et al. A machine learning approach to predict progression on active surveillance for prostate cancer. Urologic Oncology [Internet]. 2022;**40**(4):161.e1-161.e7. Available from: https://pubmed.ncbi.nlm.nih.gov/34465541/ [Accessed: June 14, 2024]

[38] Harrer S, Shah P, Antony B, Hu J. Artificial intelligence for clinical trial design. Trends in Pharmacological Sciences. 2019;**40**(8):577-591

[39] Zhang B, Zhang L, Chen Q, Jin Z, Liu S, Zhang S. Harnessing artificial intelligence to improve clinical trial design. Communications Medicine [Internet]. 2023;**3**(1):1-3. Available from: https://www.nature.com/articles/s43856-023-00425-3 [Accessed: June 21, 2024]

[40] Singh S, Gupta H, Sharma P, Sahi S. Advances in artificial intelligence (AI)-assisted approaches in drug screening. Artificial Intelligence Chemistry. 2024;**2**(1):100039

[41] Yang S, Kar S. Application of artificial intelligence and machine learning in early detection of adverse drug reactions (ADRs) and drug-induced toxicity. Artificial Intelligence Chemistry. 2023;**1**(2):100011

[42] Ietswaart R, Arat S, Chen AX, Farahmand S, Kim B, DuMouchel W, et al. Machine learning guided association of adverse drug reactions with in vitro target-based pharmacology. EBioMedicine [Internet]. 2020;**57**. Available from: http://www.thelancet.com/article/S2352396420302127/fulltext [Accessed: June 21, 2024]

[43] Litvinova O, Yeung AWK, Hammerle FP, Mickael ME, Matin M, Kletecka-Pulker M, et al. Digital technology applications in the management of adverse drug reactions: Bibliometric analysis. Pharmaceuticals [Internet]. 2024;**17**:395. Available from: https://www.mdpi.com/1424-8247/17/3/395/htm [Accessed: June 21, 2024]

[44] Wu T, Gao CC, Lin JS, Zha JL. Active monitoring of adverse drug reactions with neural network technology. Chinese Medical Journal (Engl) [Internet]. 2017;**130**(12):1498. Available from: https://pmc/articles/PMC5463482/ [Accessed: June 21, 2024]

[45] Askin S, Burkhalter D, Calado G, El Dakrouni S. Artificial intelligence applied to clinical trials: Opportunities and challenges. Health and Technology (Berl) [Internet]. 2023;**13**(2):203. Available from: https://pmc/articles/PMC9974218/ [Accessed: June 21, 2024]

[46] Yang F, Zhang Q, Ji X, Zhang Y, Li W, Peng S, et al. Machine learning

applications in drug repurposing. Interdisciplinary Sciences [Internet]. 2022;**14**(1):15. Available from: https://pmc/articles/PMC8783773/ [Accessed: June 21, 2024]

[47] Yan C, Grabowska ME, Dickson AL, Li B, Wen Z, Roden DM, et al. Leveraging generative AI to prioritize drug repurposing candidates for Alzheimer's disease with real-world clinical validation. npj Digital Medicine [Internet]. 2024;**7**(1):1-6. Available from: https://www.nature.com/articles/s41746-024-01038-3 [Accessed: June 21, 2024]

[48] Paul D, Sanap G, Shenoy S, Kalyane D, Kalia K, Tekade RK. Artificial intelligence in drug discovery and development. Drug Discovery Today [Internet]. 2021;**26**(1):80. Available from: https://pmc/articles/PMC7577280/ [Accessed: June 21, 2024]

[49] Huang JY, Lee WP, Der LK. Predicting adverse drug reactions from social media posts: Data balance, feature selection and deep learning. Healthcare [Internet]. 2022;**10**(4). Available from: https://pmc/articles/PMC9024774/ [Accessed: June 4, 2024]

[50] Alowais SA, Alghamdi SS, Alsuhebany N, Alqahtani T, Alshaya AI, Almohareb SN, et al. Revolutionizing healthcare: The role of artificial intelligence in clinical practice. BMC Medical Education [Internet]. 2023;**23**(1). Available from: https://pmc/articles/PMC10517477/ [Accessed: June 4, 2024]

Chapter 3

The Impact of Technological Progress on Pharmacovigilance

Jian Yang and Fan Li

Abstract

The rapid advancement of technology, particularly in Artificial Intelligence (AI), Machine Learning (ML), and Big Data analytics, has significantly transformed the field of pharmacovigilance. These technologies have revolutionized how adverse drug reactions (ADRs) are detected, assessed, and managed, leading to more efficient, accurate, and proactive pharmacovigilance systems. This chapter provides an analysis of the impact of AI and ML on pharmacovigilance, highlighting their roles in enhancing data collection and analysis, improving safety signal identification, and increasing the accuracy and timeliness of adverse event reporting. Additionally, it discusses the application of generative AI in natural language processing (NLP) for analyzing large datasets and generating human-like text based on learned patterns. The chapter also addresses both the benefits and risks associated with these technologies. While randomized clinical trials are essential for establishing the safety and efficacy of pharmaceutical products, they do not guarantee complete safety under all circumstances. Consequently, biopharmaceutical companies are increasingly adopting these advanced technologies to systematically detect, assess, understand, and prevent ADRs. Despite significant advantages—such as automated screening of large datasets and improved identification of safety issues—challenges related to data quality, algorithmic transparency, and regulatory compliance remain critical considerations for the future of pharmacovigilance.

Keywords: pharmacovigilance, artificial intelligence, machine learning, big data analysis, adverse drug reactions, drug safety, healthcare technology

1. Introduction

Pharmacovigilance, the scientific discipline concerned with the detection, assessment, understanding, and prevention of adverse effects or any other drug-related problems, is fundamental to ensuring the safety of medications throughout their lifecycle [1]. Traditional pharmacovigilance methods, which largely depend on spontaneous reporting systems, have provided essential insights into drug safety [2]. However, these conventional approaches are often limited by the sheer volume and complexity of data, as well as by delays in signal detection and response times [3].

These limitations can lead to significant safety risks, especially when emerging adverse drug reactions (ADRs) are not identified and addressed promptlyent years, technological advancements, particularly in artificial intelligence (AI) and machine learning (ML), have introduced new opportunities to enhance pharmacovigilance practices [4]. AI and ML offer sophisticated tools for analyzing large and complex datasets, which traditional methods may struggle to handle effectively [5]. By automating data collection and processing, these technologies can reduce the time and effort required to identify safety signals, thereby increasing the accuracy and timeliness of adverse event reporting [6].

AI anologies are particularly valuable in improving the identification of safety signals from diverse data sources, including electronic health records (EHRs), social media, and patient registries [7]. These technologies can integrate and analyze data from various formats—structured, semi-structured, and unstructured—offering a more comprehensive view of drug safety [8]. For instance, natural language processing (NLP), a subset of AI, can extract relevant information from unstructured text data such as clinical notes and social media posts, significantly expanding the scope and accuracy of pharmacovigilance activities [9].

Moreover, AI-based predictive analytics in pharmacovigilance, allowing for the early detection of potential ADRs even before they manifest in the general population. By leveraging historical data, these technologies can predict which patient populations are at higher risk for specific ADRs, facilitating more personalized and proactive interventions. This predictive capability is particularly valuable during the post-marketing surveillance phase, where ongoing monitoring of drug safety is critical [10].

Despite these advancements of AI and ML into pharmacovigilance are not without challenges [11], issues related to data quality, algorithmic transparency, and regulatory compliance must be carefully managed to realize the full potential of these technologies [12]. Ensuring high-quality, consistent data is crucial for training accurate and reliable AI models, while transparency in algorithmic decision-making is necessary to maintain trust among healthcare professionals and regulatory bodies [13].

This chapter delves informative impact of AI and ML on pharmacovigilance, examining their applications in data integration, signal detection, and predictive analytics. It also discusses the challenges associated with the adoption of these technologies and explores future directions for the field. By integrating AI and ML, pharmacovigilance systems can become more proactive and effective, ultimately enhancing drug safety and improving patient outcomes in an increasingly complex healthcare landscape.

1.1 Artificial intelligence and machine learning (ML)

1.1.1 Overview of AI and ML in pharmacovigilance

Artificial Intelligence (AI) and Machine Learning (ML) are advanced computational techniques designed to replicate tasks that typically require human intelligence, such as pattern recognition, decision-making, and predictive analytics [14]. In the context of pharmacovigilance, AI and ML are primarily employed in natural language processing (NLP) and machine learning applications, enabling the systematic analysis of large datasets to identify and manage adverse drug reactions (ADRs) [15]. These technologies offer a significant advantage in managing and analyzing large volumes of complex data, which traditional methods often struggle to handle effectively.

The methodology employed in this study integrates multiple facets of AI and ML to enhance various pharmacovigilance activities. The approach begins with data collection and preprocessing, utilizing a diverse range of data sources, including electronic health records (EHRs), social media, clinical trial data, and spontaneous reporting systems [16]. These data sources are processed using NLP techniques, particularly generative AI, which is designed to understand and generate human-like text based on patterns learned from large datasets. This capability allows for the extraction of relevant information from unstructured data sources such as clinical narratives and social media posts, significantly broadening the scope of pharmacovigilance activities and enabling the identification of ADRs from previously underutilized sources [17].

AI and ML algorithms are applied to these heterogeneous data sources, efficiently processing and integrating them to provide a more comprehensive understanding of drug safety. The models developed in this study are validated through rigorous testing procedures, including cross-validation and sensitivity analyses, to ensure their reliability and generalizability. These models are specifically leveraged for signal detection, data mining, and predictive analytics, providing a detailed and systematic approach to enhancing pharmacovigilance practices [18].

Moreover, the study also addresses the ethical and regulatory challenges associated with the implementation of these technologies. Emphasizing the importance of transparency, data quality, and compliance with regulatory standards, the chapter discusses the implications of using AI and ML in a field as sensitive as pharmacovigilance. This holistic approach ensures that the technological advancements not only improve the efficiency and accuracy of pharmacovigilance but also adhere to the necessary ethical guidelines and regulatory requirements [19].

By merging advanced AI and ML methodologies with comprehensive data sources and rigorous validation techniques, this study provides a robust framework for improving pharmacovigilance practices. This integrated methodology demonstrates how AI and ML can be effectively harnessed to enhance the detection and management of adverse drug reactions, ultimately contributing to safer pharmaceutical practices and better patient outcomes.

1.1.1.1 Data collection and preprocessing

- *Data sources:* The study utilized diverse data sources, including electronic health records (EHRs), social media platforms, clinical trial data, and spontaneous reporting systems. Each of these data sources provides unique insights into drug safety, with EHRs offering structured clinical data, social media providing unstructured patient-reported outcomes, and clinical trial data contributing pre-market safety information [20].

- *Data preprocessing:* Given the variety of data formats, the preprocessing phase involved cleaning and standardizing the data to ensure consistency and accuracy. Structured data, such as that from EHRs, was normalized and encoded, while unstructured data from social media was processed using natural language processing (NLP) techniques. NLP was employed to extract relevant entities such as drug names, symptoms, and adverse events from free-text data, which was then structured for further analysis.

1.1.1.2 Signal detection

- *Application of ML algorithms:* For signal detection, machine learning algorithms such as Random Forests, Support Vector Machines (SVM), and Gradient Boosting Machines were implemented. These algorithms were trained on historical data to identify patterns and correlations that could indicate potential safety signals. The models were validated using cross-validation techniques to ensure robustness and generalizability across different datasets [21].

- *NLP for unstructured data:* In addition to structured data analysis, NLP techniques were applied to unstructured data sources like social media and clinical notes. Named entity recognition (NER) and sentiment analysis were used to detect mentions of adverse events and assess the sentiment associated with these mentions. The integration of NLP with traditional ML models enhanced the detection of emerging safety signals from non-traditional data sources [22].

1.1.1.3 Predictive analytics

- *Predictive modeling:* The study also focused on predictive analytics, using ML models to forecast the likelihood of adverse drug reactions (ADRs) in specific patient populations. Predictive models were developed using historical ADR data and patient demographics, enabling the identification of high-risk groups. Techniques such as logistic regression and deep learning were employed to build these models, with performance metrics like precision, recall, and the area under the receiver operating characteristic (ROC) curve used to evaluate their effectiveness [23].

- *Real-time data processing:* To facilitate timely decision-making, real-time data processing capabilities were integrated into the pharmacovigilance system. Streaming data from EHRs and social media was continuously fed into the ML models, allowing for the real-time detection of potential safety issues. This proactive approach enabled quicker regulatory responses and improved patient safety outcomes [24].

1.1.1.4 Model validation and interpretation:

- *Validation techniques:* Rigorous validation techniques were applied to ensure the reliability of the AI and ML models. This included splitting the data into training, validation, and test sets, and using techniques such as k-fold cross-validation to minimize overfitting. The models were also subjected to sensitivity analyses to understand the impact of various input features on the predictions.

- *Interpretability of models:* To address concerns about the "black box" nature of AI models, methods such as SHAP (SHapley Additive exPlanations) and LIME (Local Interpretable Model-agnostic Explanations) were employed to provide interpretability. These techniques allowed for the identification of key variables that influenced the model's predictions, thereby increasing the transparency and trustworthiness of the AI-driven pharmacovigilance processes [25].

1.1.1.5 Data integration and reporting

- *Integration of data sources:* The integration of multiple data sources was critical for a holistic view of drug safety. Data integration frameworks were developed to merge structured and unstructured data, ensuring that the output from one model could be effectively used as input for another. This seamless integration allowed for comprehensive analysis and reporting [26].

- *Automated reporting:* The findings from the AI and ML models were used to generate automated reports, which were then reviewed by pharmacovigilance professionals for final validation. These reports provided actionable insights, including the identification of new safety signals, risk predictions, and recommendations for regulatory actions.

This methodology highlights the sophisticated application of AI and ML in pharmacovigilance, demonstrating how these technologies can enhance data analysis, signal detection, and predictive capabilities. The systematic approach to data collection, model development, validation, and integration ensures that the pharmacovigilance process is both rigorous and scalable, ultimately contributing to improved drug safety and patient outcomes.

By systematically applying these research methods, this chapter provides a robust analysis of how AI and ML technologies can transform pharmacovigilance practices. The combination of theoretical insights, practical applications, and ethical considerations offers a comprehensive view of the opportunities and challenges in this evolving field.

1.1.2 Applications in pharmacovigilance

AI and ML are increasingly being used to enhance various pharmacovigilance activities. For instance, ML algorithms can analyze EHRs, social media posts, and other data sources to identify potential ADRs. Deep learning, a subset of ML, has shown particular promise in improving the accuracy and efficiency of these analyses. According to Evans HP et al. [27], deep learning models can significantly enhance the detection of ADRs by analyzing complex datasets more effectively than traditional statistical methods [27].

One notable application is in signal detection, where AI and ML algorithms can sift through vast datasets to identify new safety signals. This proactive approach can lead to earlier identification of potential drug safety issues, enabling quicker regulatory actions and mitigating risks to patients. For example, AI-driven signal detection systems can continuously monitor and analyze data from various sources, providing real-time updates on potential safety concerns.

Another significant application is in the prediction of ADRs. By leveraging historical data, ML models can predict the likelihood of ADRs for new drugs or new patient populations. This predictive capability is particularly valuable during the early stages of drug development, where understanding the safety profile of a drug is crucial. Predictive models can also be used to identify patient subgroups at higher risk of ADRs, enabling more personalized and safer medication regimens [28].

Furthermore, AI and ML can assist in automating routine pharmacovigilance tasks such as case processing and report generation. Automation can significantly reduce the workload on pharmacovigilance professionals, allowing them to focus on more complex and value-added activities. For instance, NLP algorithms can automatically extract relevant information from adverse event reports, classify the events, and generate comprehensive reports, thereby streamlining the entire pharmacovigilance workflow.

1.1.3 Benefits and challenges

The integration of AI and ML in pharmacovigilance offers numerous benefits, including increased efficiency, accuracy, and the ability to handle large and complex datasets. These technologies can reduce the time required for data analysis, allowing for real-time monitoring and quicker response to potential safety issues. Moreover, AI and ML can uncover hidden patterns and correlations, providing deeper insights into drug safety.

AI and ML also have the potential to improve the consistency and standardization of pharmacovigilance processes. By automating routine tasks and providing consistent analyses, these technologies can reduce human errors and variability, leading to more reliable and reproducible results. Additionally, AI and ML can facilitate the integration of pharmacovigilance data with other healthcare data sources, such as clinical trials and genomics data, enabling a more holistic approach to drug safety monitoring [29].

However, there are challenges associated with the implementation of AI and ML in pharmacovigilance. Data quality and consistency are critical for the accuracy of AI models. Poor quality or inconsistent data can lead to biased or inaccurate results, undermining the reliability of AI-driven analyses. Ensuring data quality requires robust data governance frameworks, including standardized data collection and processing procedures, as well as ongoing monitoring and validation of data sources.

Additionally, there are concerns regarding the transparency and interpretability of AI algorithms, often referred to as the "black box" problem. AI models, particularly deep learning models, can be highly complex and difficult to interpret, making it challenging to understand how they arrive at their conclusions. This lack of transparency can hinder the acceptance and trust of AI-driven approaches among regulatory authorities and healthcare professionals [30].

Regulatory acceptance of AI-driven approaches also remains a significant hurdle. The regulatory landscape for AI in pharmacovigilance is still evolving, and there is a need for clear guidelines and validation processes to ensure the reliability and robustness of these technologies. Regulators must balance the potential benefits of AI with the need to protect patient safety and maintain public trust in the healthcare system. Collaborative efforts between regulators, industry, and academia are essential to develop and implement appropriate regulatory frameworks for AI in pharmacovigilance.

1.2 Big data analysis

1.2.1 Introduction to big data in pharmacovigilance

Big Data refers to large, complex datasets that cannot be easily managed or analyzed using traditional data processing techniques. In pharmacovigilance, Big Data encompasses diverse sources, including electronic health records (EHRs), clinical trial data, social media, patient registries, and spontaneous reporting systems. The ability to analyze these vast datasets in real-time offers significant advantages in detecting and managing adverse drug reactions (ADRs) [31].

Big Data in the context of pharmacovigilance is characterized by its volume, velocity, variety, and veracity. The volume refers to the enormous amount of data generated daily from multiple sources. For instance, EHRs alone generate vast amounts of patient data, including diagnosis, medication, treatment outcomes, and more. Velocity pertains to the speed at which this data is generated and needs to be processed. With real-time health monitoring and reporting systems, data is constantly being updated, necessitating rapid processing capabilities [32].

Variety highlights the different forms of data—structured data from clinical trials, semi-structured data from EHRs, and unstructured data from social media and patient forums. Each of these data types requires different methods of processing and analysis. Veracity refers to the reliability and accuracy of the data. Ensuring the data's integrity and consistency is critical for meaningful analysis and decision-making.

In pharmacovigilance, Big Data's significance cannot be overstated. Traditional pharmacovigilance relied heavily on spontaneous reporting systems and clinical trial data, which, while valuable, often provided limited insights due to the smaller datasets and reporting biases. Big Data allows for the integration of multiple data sources, providing a more comprehensive view of drug safety. For example, social media platforms and patient forums can offer real-time insights into patient experiences and emerging safety concerns that might not be captured through traditional reporting systems [33].

1.2.2 Utilization of big data in drug safety

Big Data analytics involves the use of advanced data processing tools and techniques to analyze large volumes of data and extract meaningful insights. In pharmacovigilance, Big Data analytics can significantly improve the detection of ADRs, enhance risk management, and support regulatory decision-making. By integrating various data sources, pharmacovigilance systems can achieve a more comprehensive view of drug safety [34].

One of the primary benefits of Big Data in pharmacovigilance is the enhanced ability to detect ADRs. Traditional methods of ADR detection often rely on healthcare professionals to report suspected reactions, which can lead to underreporting and delays in identifying safety issues. Big Data analytics can process vast amounts of data from various sources, including EHRs, clinical trial data, and social media, to identify patterns and trends indicative of ADRs.

For example, machine learning algorithms can be employed to analyze social media posts and detect signals of potential ADRs based on keywords and sentiment analysis. By combining data from multiple sources, including patient registries and EHRs, it is possible to validate these signals and gain a more accurate understanding of a drug's safety profile. This holistic approach enables earlier detection of safety signals and more proactive risk management [35].

Big Data analytics also supports regulatory decision-making by providing comprehensive insights into drug safety. Regulatory agencies such as the FDA and EMA can use Big Data to monitor post-market drug safety and evaluate the risk-benefit profiles of medications. By integrating data from clinical trials, EHRs, and spontaneous reporting systems, regulatory bodies can make more informed decisions regarding drug approvals, labeling changes, and market withdrawals [36].

Moreover, Big Data can facilitate the identification of subpopulations at higher risk of ADRs. For instance, data from EHRs can be used to analyze the effects of a drug in different demographic groups such as age, gender, and comorbidities. This information can inform targeted risk mitigation strategies and improve patient safety.

1.2.3 Challenges and future directions

Despite the potential benefits, the utilization of Big Data in pharmacovigilance presents several challenges. Data integration from diverse sources requires standardization and interoperability to ensure consistent and accurate analysis. Privacy and security concerns also arise with the handling of sensitive health data, necessitating robust data protection measures.

One of the significant challenges in utilizing Big Data for pharmacovigilance is data integration. Data from different sources often come in various formats and structures, making it difficult to combine and analyze them cohesively. For instance, EHRs from different healthcare providers may use different coding systems and terminologies, while social media data is unstructured and requires advanced natural language processing techniques to extract relevant information [37].

Standardization is crucial to address these challenges. Developing common data standards and protocols can facilitate the integration of diverse data sources and improve data interoperability. Initiatives such as the Observational Medical Outcomes Partnership (OMOP) and the Sentinel System are working towards creating standardized data models and vocabularies to support Big Data analytics in healthcare.

The handling of sensitive health data raises significant privacy and security concerns. Big Data analytics in pharmacovigilance involves processing large volumes of personal health information, which must be protected to ensure patient confidentiality. Ensuring compliance with data protection regulations such as the General Data Protection Regulation (GDPR) in Europe and the Health Insurance Portability and Accountability Act (HIPAA) in the United States is essential [38].

Implementing robust data encryption, access controls, and anonymization techniques can help mitigate privacy and security risks. Additionally, developing policies and frameworks for ethical data use is critical to maintaining public trust and ensuring the responsible use of Big Data in pharmacovigilance.

Looking ahead, the integration of artificial intelligence (AI) and machine learning (ML) with Big Data analytics holds promise for further advancements in pharmacovigilance. AI and ML can enhance the predictive capabilities of pharmacovigilance systems, enabling earlier detection of ADRs and more efficient risk management. For example, predictive models can be developed to identify patients at high risk of experiencing ADRs based on their medical history, genetic information, and other factors [39].

Furthermore, the development of more sophisticated algorithms and computational models can improve the accuracy and reliability of Big Data analytics. Advances in natural language processing and sentiment analysis can enhance the ability to extract meaningful insights from unstructured data sources such as social media and patient forums.

In conclusion, while the utilization of Big Data in pharmacovigilance presents challenges, the potential benefits are significant. By addressing issues related to data integration, privacy, and security, and leveraging advanced analytics techniques, pharmacovigilance systems can achieve a more comprehensive and accurate understanding of drug safety. The integration of AI and ML with Big Data analytics holds promise for further advancements, ultimately leading to better patient outcomes and improved public health.

2. Case studies and data analysis

2.1 Case study: AI in signal detection

2.1.1 Introduction to AI in signal detection

Artificial Intelligence (AI) has significantly impacted various sectors, including healthcare. In the realm of pharmacovigilance, AI is used for signal detection, particularly in identifying adverse drug reactions (ADRs). This section explores the application of deep learning models in enhancing pharmacovigilance, illustrating how large datasets and advanced algorithms can improve the identification and monitoring of ADRs, thereby enhancing patient safety and regulatory decisions [40].

2.1.2 Deep learning models for signal detection in healthcare

2.1.2.1 Data sources and preparation

The foundation of effective AI in signal detection is a robust dataset. For instance, a comprehensive dataset might include over one million patient records spanning 5 years. Such a dataset typically comprises patient demographics, medication histories, clinical notes, and laboratory results. These diverse data types provide a rich source of information for training deep learning models (**Table 1**).

2.1.2.2 Model selection and training

Deep learning models like convolutional neural networks (CNNs) and recurrent neural networks (RNNs) are particularly effective for this task. CNNs are adept at handling structured data such as demographics and medication histories, while RNNs excel with sequential data, including clinical notes and laboratory results (**Table 2**).

2.1.2.3 Real-time application

Once trained, these models can be deployed to process new data in real-time, identifying potential ADRs as they occur. This real-time capability is crucial for prompt detection and response to emerging drug safety issues.

2.1.3 Results and findings

Deep learning models have demonstrated substantial effectiveness in ADR detection. For instance, models can identify previously unrecognized ADRs, including rare

Step	Description
Data cleaning	Removing or imputing missing values to ensure completeness.
Standardization	Converting data into a consistent format to facilitate analysis.
Encoding	Transforming categorical variables into numerical formats that models can process.

Table 1.
Data preparation steps for deep learning models.

Process	Description
Data splitting	Dividing the dataset into training, validation, and test sets to ensure unbiased evaluation of model performance.
Model training	Utilizing historical ADR data to teach the models to recognize patterns and associations.
Hyperparameter tuning	Adjusting model parameters to optimize performance and prevent overfitting.
Model evaluation	Assessing performance using metrics like precision, recall, and F1 score on the test set.

Table 2.
Model selection and training steps for deep learning models.

and severe reactions. An example of this might include discovering a novel association between a common antihypertensive drug and a rare but serious kidney condition. Such findings are typically validated through clinical review to ensure accuracy (**Table 3**).

2.1.4 Advantages of AI in pharmacovigilance

The integration of AI and Big Data analytics in pharmacovigilance provides several key benefits:

Enhanced ADR detection: AI models can efficiently and accurately identify ADRs by recognizing patterns and anomalies that might be missed by traditional methods. This capability is particularly valuable for detecting rare or delayed ADRs.

Real-time monitoring: AI enables continuous, real-time analysis of incoming data, allowing for the swift identification of emerging safety signals. This proactive monitoring can lead to quicker regulatory actions and improved patient outcomes.

Comprehensive data integration: AI models can integrate diverse data sources such as EHRs, clinical trials, and social media. This comprehensive approach provides a more holistic view of drug safety, enhancing the robustness of signal detection.

2.1.5 Challenges and considerations

Despite its potential, the application of AI in pharmacovigilance faces several challenges:

Data quality and standardization: Ensuring consistent and high-quality data from various sources is essential. Inconsistent data formats and missing information can significantly hinder model performance. Effective data cleaning and standardization are crucial for maximizing the accuracy and reliability of AI models.

Metric	Value
Precision	0.92
Recall	0.88
F1 score	0.90
Novel ADRs identified	Multiple, including rare conditions

Table 3.
Performance metrics of deep learning models in ADR detection.

Privacy and security: Handling sensitive health data requires robust privacy and security measures to protect patient confidentiality. Compliance with regulations such as GDPR and HIPAA is essential to maintain trust and safeguard against data breaches.

Model interpretability: Deep learning models often function as "black boxes," making it difficult to interpret their decision-making processes. Developing methods to explain model predictions is important for gaining trust from healthcare professionals and regulators. Transparency and accountability are crucial for the widespread adoption of AI in healthcare.

2.1.6 Future directions

The future of AI in pharmacovigilance is promising, with several areas for ongoing research and development:

Advanced algorithms: Developing more sophisticated algorithms, such as reinforcement learning and generative models, can further enhance ADR detection and prediction capabilities. These advanced techniques hold the potential to improve the accuracy and efficiency of pharmacovigilance systems.

Interdisciplinary collaboration: Collaboration between data scientists, clinicians, and regulatory agencies is crucial for the successful implementation of AI in pharmacovigilance. This interdisciplinary approach ensures that models are clinically relevant and regulatory compliant, fostering innovation and improving drug safety [41].

Ethical considerations: Addressing ethical concerns related to AI in healthcare, such as algorithmic bias and fairness, is essential. Ensuring that AI systems are transparent, equitable, and accountable will be key to their widespread adoption. Developing guidelines and standards for ethical AI usage in pharmacovigilance can help mitigate risks and promote responsible innovation [42].

In conclusion, AI has the potential to transform pharmacovigilance by improving ADR detection through advanced deep learning models and extensive datasets. By leveraging real-time monitoring and comprehensive data integration, AI can provide more accurate and timely insights into drug safety. While challenges related to data quality, privacy, and model interpretability remain, ongoing advancements in AI and interdisciplinary collaboration hold promise for the future of pharmacovigilance.

2.2 Case study: Big data analytics in ADR management

2.2.1 Overview of big data in pharmacovigilance

Adverse drug reactions (ADRs) are a critical concern in the pharmaceutical industry, particularly when dealing with newly approved drugs. Traditional methods of monitoring ADRs primarily involve analyzing clinical trial data and post-marketing surveillance. However, with the advent of Big Data analytics, there has been a paradigm shift in ADR management. By integrating diverse data sources such as clinical trial data, electronic health records (EHRs), and social media, researchers can now create a comprehensive safety profile for new drugs, leading to earlier detection of adverse reactions and more effective risk management [43].

2.2.2 Data sources and integration

The dataset for this case study was comprehensive, comprising three main sources:

Clinical trial data: Structured data from phase I to phase III trials detailing patient demographics, drug dosages, and recorded side effects.

Electronic health records (EHRs): A mix of structured and unstructured data from multiple healthcare providers, including patient demographics, diagnoses, treatment regimens, and outcomes.

Social media posts: Unstructured data capturing patient-reported experiences and symptoms related to the drug, gathered from various social media platforms.

Combining these diverse sources into a unified dataset was essential for a holistic analysis (**Table 4**).

2.2.3 Analytical methodologies

The study employed a multi-faceted approach to analyze the integrated dataset. The methodologies included:

Data integration: Merging structured and unstructured data from various sources to form a comprehensive dataset.

Natural language processing (NLP): NLP techniques were used to process unstructured data from social media and clinical notes, extracting relevant information such as symptoms and patient experiences.

Machine learning classifiers: Algorithms such as support vector machines and neural networks were used to detect patterns and correlations within the data, classifying and predicting adverse reactions.

Traditional statistical methods: Applied to the structured data, serving as a comparative foundation for validating machine learning results (**Table 5**).

2.2.4 Key findings

The analysis yielded several critical insights into the drug's safety profile:

Early detection of adverse reactions: Within weeks of the drug's market release, an increase in patient-reported symptoms such as severe headaches and dizziness was detected on social media. This early warning prompted further investigation.

Data source	Type of data	Key attributes
Clinical trials	Structured	Patient demographics, dosages, side effects
EHRs	Structured/unstructured	Diagnoses, treatment regimens, follow-up results
Social media	Unstructured	Patient symptoms, experiences, sentiment analysis

Table 4.
Summary of data sources for comprehensive drug safety analysis.

Technique	Application
Data integration	Merging data from different sources
Natural language processing (NLP)	Extracting relevant information from unstructured data
Machine learning classifiers	Predicting and classifying adverse reactions
Traditional statistical methods	Analyzing structured data from clinical trials and EHRs

Table 5.
Analytical methodologies in pharmacovigilance data analysis.

Validation through EHRs: The association between the drug and these adverse effects was confirmed through subsequent analysis of EHRs. This led to regulatory notifications, resulting in updated safety warnings and revised prescribing information.

Enhanced safety profile: Integrating diverse data sources allowed for a more robust safety profile, facilitating better risk management and improving patient safety measures (**Table 6**).

2.2.5 Discussion and implications

The integration of Big Data analytics in ADR management offers significant advantages. By combining structured and unstructured data, researchers can achieve a holistic view of a drug's safety profile. Early detection of adverse reactions through social media monitoring allows for timely interventions, potentially reducing risks to patient health. Validation with EHR data ensures that observed trends are corroborated by clinical evidence, enhancing the credibility and reliability of the findings [44].

However, this approach also presents challenges. Integrating data from disparate sources can be complex, requiring advanced technical capabilities and significant resources. Ensuring data privacy and security is paramount, particularly when handling sensitive patient information from EHRs and social media. Additionally, regulatory frameworks must evolve to provide clear guidelines on the use of advanced analytics in pharmacovigilance [45].

2.2.6 Conclusion and future directions

Big Data analytics significantly enhances ADR management by enabling early detection and validation of adverse reactions. The integration of clinical trial data, EHRs, and social media creates a comprehensive safety profile for new drugs, ultimately improving patient safety. Continued advancements in technology and data management practices will further refine these methods, making them an integral part of pharmacovigilance efforts. Future research should focus on addressing the technical and regulatory challenges to fully realize the potential of Big Data analytics in improving drug safety.

2.2.7 Summary table

See (**Table 7**).

2.2.8 Follow-up suggestions

Further case studies: explore additional case studies that demonstrate the application of Big Data analytics in pharmacovigilance.

Insight	Source	Impact
Early detection	Social media	Prompted further investigation
Validation	EHRs	Confirmed adverse reactions, leading to regulatory actions
Enhanced safety profile	Integrated dataset	Improved risk management and patient safety

Table 6.
Key findings from integrated data analysis in drug safety.

Aspect	Description
Data sources	Clinical trials, EHRs, social media
Analytical techniques	Data integration, NLP, machine learning, statistical methods
Key findings	Early detection, validation, enhanced safety profile
Challenges	Data integration complexity, privacy and security, regulatory frameworks
Future directions	Technological advancements, regulatory evolution

Table 7.
Summary of key aspects in integrated pharmacovigilance analysis.

Regulatory challenges: investigate the evolving regulatory challenges and frameworks supporting Big Data analytics in healthcare.

Technical innovations: analyze the technical aspects and tools used for integrating and analyzing diverse data sources for ADR management.

3. Challenges and opportunities

3.1 Data quality and consistency

The efficacy of machine learning (ML) models is intrinsically linked to the quality of the training data utilized. In the context of pharmacovigilance (PV), ensuring high-quality, representative training data presents a multifaceted challenge.

Firstly, the issue of data quality encompasses several dimensions: accuracy, completeness, timeliness, and reliability [46]. Accurate data is paramount; any inaccuracies can propagate through the model, leading to erroneous conclusions. Completeness is equally critical, as missing data can skew the model's understanding and predictions. In PV, timeliness—ensuring that data is current and reflective of the latest findings and trends—is crucial, as outdated information can misinform models, particularly in a field as dynamic as drug safety. Reliability, or the trustworthiness of data sources, ensures that the data is consistent over time and not subject to random fluctuations or biases.

Data annotation is another critical aspect. For ML models to learn effectively, data must be accurately labeled—a task often requiring expert knowledge in PV. This process is labor-intensive and subject to human error, which can introduce inconsistencies and biases. Furthermore, ensuring that datasets are representative of diverse patient populations is essential to avoid biased predictions that could affect certain demographic groups disproportionately [47].

One significant challenge in PV is dealing with unstructured data such as clinical notes, patient records, and adverse event reports. Natural language processing (NLP) techniques are employed to extract meaningful information from such unstructured data, but these techniques themselves are highly dependent on the quality and representativeness of the training data.

Moreover, bias in training data is a pervasive issue. Bias can arise from various sources, including sampling methods, data collection processes, and inherent biases in human annotations. For example, if certain adverse events are underreported in the data due to socioeconomic factors, the ML model might fail to predict these events accurately. Addressing these biases requires meticulous data preprocessing, augmentation, and validation strategies [48].

In summary, ensuring data quality and consistency in PV is a complex task that requires a comprehensive approach involving accurate, complete, timely, and reliable data, effective data annotation, and robust strategies to mitigate bias. Overcoming these challenges is crucial to harnessing the full potential of ML in PV, leading to more accurate predictions and analyses and ultimately enhancing drug safety.

3.2 Regulatory and compliance issues

The integration of artificial intelligence (AI) and machine learning (ML) into pharmacovigilance (PV) practices brings forth a myriad of regulatory and compliance challenges. As the regulatory landscape for these technologies is still evolving, there is a pressing need for clear guidelines and harmonized regulations to ensure their safe and effective use.

Currently, regulatory bodies such as the FDA, EMA, and other international organizations are in the process of developing frameworks to address the unique challenges posed by AI and ML in PV. These frameworks must strike a balance between encouraging innovation and ensuring patient safety. One of the primary challenges is the lack of standardized guidelines for the development, validation, and deployment of ML models in PV. Without such guidelines, there is a risk of inconsistent practices, which can undermine the reliability and trustworthiness of ML-driven PV systems [49].

Model validation is a critical aspect of regulatory compliance. Regulatory bodies require that ML models undergo rigorous validation to ensure their accuracy, robustness, and reliability. This involves extensive testing using diverse datasets to evaluate the model's performance across different scenarios. Additionally, continuous monitoring and post-market surveillance are essential to detect any deviations in model performance over time. However, the dynamic nature of ML models, which continuously learn and adapt from new data, poses a challenge for traditional validation methods. Regulators and industry stakeholders must collaborate to develop adaptive validation frameworks that can accommodate the evolving nature of ML models [50].

Risk management is another crucial component of regulatory compliance. The use of AI and ML in PV introduces new types of risks, including algorithmic bias, data privacy concerns, and the potential for unintended consequences. To address these risks, organizations must implement robust risk management strategies, including thorough risk assessments, regular audits, and transparent reporting mechanisms. Engaging with regulators early in the development process can help organizations identify potential regulatory hurdles and develop strategies to mitigate them [51].

Moreover, regulatory compliance extends beyond the development and deployment of ML models. Organizations must also ensure that their data practices comply with data protection regulations such as GDPR and HIPAA. This involves implementing stringent data governance policies, obtaining informed consent from patients, and ensuring the anonymization of patient data.

Engaging with regulators and adopting best practices for model validation and risk management are crucial for overcoming these regulatory challenges. By fostering a collaborative relationship with regulatory bodies, organizations can stay abreast of regulatory developments and ensure that their ML-driven PV practices align with regulatory expectations. Additionally, participating in industry forums and working groups can provide valuable insights and contribute to the development of harmonized regulations [52].

In conclusion, navigating the regulatory and compliance landscape for AI and ML in PV is a complex but essential endeavor. Clear guidelines, adaptive validation frameworks, robust risk management strategies, and proactive engagement with regulators are key to ensuring the safe and effective use of these technologies in enhancing drug safety and improving patient outcomes.

3.3 Technological integration

Integrating artificial intelligence (AI), machine learning (ML), and Big Data technologies into existing pharmacovigilance (PV) systems represents a monumental task, demanding significant investment in both infrastructure and human capital. The complexity of this integration arises from several factors, including the need for advanced computational infrastructure, data management systems, and the cultivation of a workforce proficient in these cutting-edge technologies [53].

To begin with, the existing PV infrastructure often comprises disparate systems that have evolved over time. These systems may include databases of adverse event reports, electronic health records (EHRs), clinical trial data, and other sources of health information. Integrating AI and ML technologies into these systems requires the development of sophisticated data pipelines that can seamlessly extract, transform, and load (ETL) data from multiple sources into a unified analytical framework. This process is not trivial, as it involves ensuring data compatibility, resolving discrepancies, and maintaining data integrity across diverse datasets [54].

Investing in modern computational infrastructure is a prerequisite for harnessing the power of AI and ML in PV. High-performance computing (HPC) resources, including powerful servers, data storage solutions, and network capabilities, are essential to handle the vast amounts of data involved in PV. Organizations must also consider the scalability of their infrastructure to accommodate future growth in data volume and computational demands [55].

However, technology alone is not sufficient. The successful integration of AI and ML into PV systems hinges on the skills and expertise of the workforce. Organizations must invest in comprehensive training programs to equip their staff with the necessary skills to utilize these technologies effectively. This includes training in data science, statistical analysis, programming, and the specific applications of AI and ML in PV. Moreover, fostering a culture of continuous learning and innovation is crucial, as the field of AI and ML is rapidly evolving [56].

The integration of multiple technologies to create a seamless workflow presents additional challenges. For instance, combining AI algorithms with Big Data analytics requires careful orchestration to ensure that the output of one system can be effectively utilized by another. This involves the development of interoperability standards and protocols that facilitate the smooth exchange of data and insights between different systems. Additionally, the implementation of AI-driven PV systems must be accompanied by robust validation and testing processes to ensure their reliability and accuracy [57].

One significant aspect of technological integration is the implementation of real-time data processing capabilities. In traditional PV systems, data analysis often occurs in batch mode, with periodic updates. However, the integration of AI and Big Data technologies enables real-time monitoring and analysis of adverse events. This shift towards real-time PV can significantly enhance the responsiveness and effectiveness of drug safety monitoring, allowing for quicker identification and mitigation of potential risks.

Moreover, the integration of AI and ML into PV systems can facilitate predictive analytics, enabling proactive identification of potential safety issues before they manifest as adverse events. By analyzing patterns and trends in historical data, AI algorithms can predict future risks and provide early warnings, allowing for timely interventions. This proactive approach represents a significant advancement over traditional reactive PV methods.

Another critical aspect of technological integration is the collaboration between various stakeholders, including healthcare providers, regulatory agencies, pharmaceutical companies, and technology vendors. Effective collaboration is essential to ensure that AI and ML technologies are implemented in a manner that aligns with regulatory requirements and industry best practices. Collaborative initiatives, such as data sharing agreements and joint research projects, can also enhance the quality and scope of data available for PV, further improving the performance of AI-driven systems [58].

In conclusion, the integration of AI, ML, and Big Data technologies into PV systems presents both significant challenges and opportunities. By investing in advanced infrastructure, fostering a skilled workforce, and facilitating seamless interoperability between technologies, organizations can harness the full potential of these innovations to enhance drug safety monitoring. As AI and ML continue to evolve, their integration into PV systems will undoubtedly transform the field, making it more proactive, efficient, and effective.

3.4 Future directions

The future of pharmacovigilance (PV) is poised for significant transformation, driven by the continued advancement and integration of artificial intelligence (AI), machine learning (ML), and Big Data technologies. These innovations promise to enhance drug safety monitoring, improve patient outcomes, and usher in a new era of proactive and efficient PV practices.

One of the most exciting future directions in PV is the development of more sophisticated AI and ML algorithms. These algorithms will be capable of analyzing vast amounts of data with unprecedented accuracy and speed. For instance, deep learning models, which mimic the neural networks of the human brain, can identify complex patterns and relationships within the data that traditional statistical methods might overlook. These advanced algorithms can improve the detection of adverse drug reactions (ADRs), predict potential safety issues, and provide actionable insights for healthcare providers and regulatory agencies [59].

Improving data quality and integration will also play a crucial role in the future of PV. As AI and ML models are only as good as the data they are trained on, efforts to enhance data collection, curation, and annotation will be paramount. This includes developing standardized protocols for data reporting and ensuring that datasets are representative of diverse patient populations. Enhanced data integration techniques will allow for the seamless combination of structured and unstructured data from various sources such as EHRs, clinical trials, social media, and patient registries. This comprehensive approach to data management will enable more holistic and accurate analyses [60].

The future of PV will also be characterized by increased collaboration between stakeholders. Pharmaceutical companies, regulatory agencies, healthcare providers, and technology vendors will need to work together to develop and implement AI-driven PV systems. Collaborative efforts, such as public-private partnerships and industry consortia, can facilitate the sharing of data, resources, and expertise, ultimately leading to more robust and effective PV practices. Additionally, international collaboration will be essential to harmonize regulations and standards, ensuring the safe and consistent use of AI and ML technologies across different regions.

Regulatory frameworks will continue to evolve to keep pace with technological advancements. Regulators will need to develop adaptive and flexible guidelines that can accommodate the dynamic nature of AI and ML models. This includes establishing criteria for model validation, monitoring, and risk management, as well as addressing ethical considerations related to data privacy, transparency, and accountability. Proactive engagement with regulators will be crucial for organizations to navigate the complex regulatory landscape and ensure compliance [61].

Ethical considerations will also play a pivotal role in shaping the future of PV. As AI and ML technologies become more prevalent, it is essential to address issues related to data privacy, algorithmic bias, and transparency. Ensuring that AI-driven PV systems are fair, unbiased, and transparent will be critical to maintaining public trust and confidence. This includes implementing rigorous ethical guidelines, conducting regular audits, and fostering a culture of accountability within organizations.

The integration of emerging technologies such as blockchain and the Internet of Things (IoT) will further enhance PV practices. Blockchain technology can provide a secure and transparent way to record and share data, ensuring the integrity and traceability of PV records. IoT devices, such as wearable health monitors, can provide real-time data on patient health and drug effects, enabling continuous and proactive monitoring of drug safety [62].

Looking ahead, the role of patient engagement and empowerment will become increasingly important in PV. AI-driven platforms can facilitate patient involvement by providing user-friendly interfaces for reporting ADRs, accessing personalized drug safety information, and participating in post-marketing surveillance studies. Empowering patients to take an active role in PV can lead to more comprehensive and accurate data collection, ultimately improving drug safety outcomes [63].

In conclusion, the future of pharmacovigilance lies in the continued advancement and integration of AI, ML, and Big Data technologies. By developing more sophisticated algorithms, improving data quality and integration, fostering collaboration between stakeholders, and addressing ethical considerations, the field of PV will evolve into a more proactive, efficient, and effective discipline. These advancements will not only enhance drug safety monitoring but also contribute to better patient outcomes and a more resilient healthcare system.

3.5 Ethical considerations

As artificial intelligence (AI) and machine learning (ML) technologies become increasingly integrated into pharmacovigilance (PV), ethical considerations have emerged as a critical focal point. Ensuring that AI-driven PV systems operate in a manner that is ethical, transparent, and respectful of patient privacy is essential to maintaining public trust and maximizing the benefits of these technologies. This section explores the key ethical issues in AI and ML for PV, including data privacy, algorithmic bias, transparency, and accountability [64].

3.5.1 Data privacy

Data privacy is a paramount concern in the use of AI and ML for PV. These technologies rely on vast amounts of data, often including sensitive patient information.

Ensuring the privacy and security of this data is crucial to prevent unauthorized access, data breaches, and potential misuse. Regulations such as the General Data Protection Regulation (GDPR) in Europe and the Health Insurance Portability and Accountability Act (HIPAA) in the United States set stringent requirements for data protection [65].

Organizations must implement robust data governance frameworks that encompass data encryption, anonymization, and access controls. Encryption ensures that data is secure both in transit and at rest, while anonymization techniques remove personally identifiable information, reducing the risk of patient re-identification. Access controls limit data access to authorized personnel only, minimizing the potential for data breaches.

Moreover, obtaining informed consent from patients is a critical ethical requirement. Patients should be fully aware of how their data will be used, the purposes of the data collection, and their rights regarding data privacy. Transparent communication and clear consent processes help build trust and ensure compliance with ethical and legal standards [66].

3.5.2 Algorithmic bias

Algorithmic bias is another significant ethical concern in AI and ML for PV. Bias in algorithms can arise from various sources, including biased training data, flawed model design, and biased decision-making processes. Such biases can lead to unfair and potentially harmful outcomes, particularly for underrepresented or vulnerable populations.

To mitigate algorithmic bias, it is essential to ensure that training datasets are representative of diverse patient populations. This involves including data from different demographic groups, geographic regions, and clinical settings. Additionally, rigorous testing and validation processes should be employed to detect and address biases in AI models. Techniques such as fairness-aware machine learning and bias correction algorithms can be used to enhance the fairness and equity of AI-driven PV systems [67].

Transparency in model development and deployment is also crucial for addressing algorithmic bias. Organizations should document and disclose the sources of data, the methods used for data preprocessing and model training, and the criteria for model evaluation. This transparency allows for independent audits and assessments, promoting accountability and trust.

3.5.3 Transparency

Transparency extends beyond addressing algorithmic bias; it encompasses the entire lifecycle of AI and ML systems. Transparent AI systems are those whose decision-making processes can be understood and scrutinized by stakeholders, including healthcare providers, regulators, and patients. This is particularly important in PV, where AI-driven decisions can have significant implications for drug safety and patient health [68].

Explainable AI (XAI) techniques are designed to make AI models more transparent and interpretable. These techniques provide insights into how models make decisions, the factors influencing those decisions, and the potential limitations of the models. By making AI systems more transparent, XAI helps ensure that stakeholders can understand and trust the outputs of AI-driven PV systems [69].

In addition to technical transparency, organizational transparency is also important. Organizations should establish clear policies and procedures for the development, deployment, and monitoring of AI and ML systems. Regular reporting on AI activities, including performance metrics, risk assessments, and ethical considerations, helps maintain transparency and accountability.

3.5.4 Accountability

Accountability is a fundamental ethical principle that requires organizations to take responsibility for the actions and outcomes of their AI and ML systems. In the context of PV, this means ensuring that AI-driven systems are used in a manner that prioritizes patient safety and adheres to ethical standards.

To achieve accountability, organizations should implement comprehensive governance frameworks that define roles and responsibilities for AI activities. These frameworks should include mechanisms for monitoring and auditing AI systems, identifying and addressing potential ethical issues, and ensuring compliance with regulatory requirements [70].

Moreover, organizations should establish clear lines of accountability for decision-making processes involving AI. This includes defining who is responsible for the development, validation, and deployment of AI models, as well as who is accountable for the outcomes of AI-driven decisions. By establishing clear accountability structures, organizations can ensure that ethical considerations are prioritized throughout the lifecycle of AI systems.

3.5.5 Ethical training and culture

Finally, fostering an ethical culture within organizations is essential for addressing the ethical challenges of AI and ML in PV. This involves providing training and education on ethical principles, data privacy, algorithmic fairness, and transparency. By raising awareness and promoting ethical practices, organizations can ensure that their staff are equipped to navigate the complex ethical landscape of AI-driven PV.

Creating a culture of ethics also requires leadership commitment and organizational support. Leaders should champion ethical principles, establish clear ethical guidelines, and encourage open dialog on ethical issues. By embedding ethics into the organizational culture, organizations can ensure that ethical considerations are integral to their AI and ML initiatives [71].

In conclusion, addressing ethical considerations is crucial for the successful integration of AI and ML in pharmacovigilance. By prioritizing data privacy, mitigating algorithmic bias, ensuring transparency, establishing accountability, and fostering an ethical culture, organizations can harness the full potential of AI and ML to enhance drug safety monitoring while maintaining public trust and adhering to ethical standards.

4. Case studies

4.1 Predictive modeling for adverse drug reactions

A notable case study involves the use of machine learning (ML) algorithms to predict adverse drug reactions (ADRs) before they occur. A large pharmaceutical company implemented a predictive modeling system that analyzed historical clinical trial data, electronic health records (EHRs), and patient demographics to identify potential ADRs [72].

4.1.1 Results

The predictive model significantly improved the accuracy of ADR detection compared to traditional methods. This allowed the company to proactively address potential safety issues, reducing the incidence of ADRs and enhancing patient safety. Moreover, the insights gained from the model helped inform the design of future clinical trials, making them safer and more efficient.

4.1.2 Lessons learned

The importance of high-quality, representative data for training ML models cannot be overstated. Ensuring that the datasets used are comprehensive and inclusive of diverse patient populations is critical for the model's effectiveness. Continuous monitoring and updating of the model to incorporate new data and adapt to emerging trends are also essential. Additionally, integrating predictive analytics into existing pharmacovigilance workflows can significantly enhance drug safety by enabling early intervention and risk mitigation [73].

4.2 Natural language processing for adverse event reporting

Another successful application of AI in pharmacovigilance is the use of natural language processing (NLP) to analyze adverse event reports. A regulatory agency implemented an NLP system to process the vast number of adverse event reports it receives annually. Traditionally, these reports were manually reviewed by pharmacovigilance experts, a time-consuming and labor-intensive process.

4.2.1 Results

The NLP system was designed to extract relevant information from unstructured text, such as symptoms, drug names, dosages, and patient demographics [74]. By automating the initial review process, the system significantly reduced the workload of pharmacovigilance experts, allowing them to focus on more complex cases. The NLP system also improved the consistency and accuracy of data extraction, leading to more reliable adverse event monitoring.

4.2.2 Lessons learned

The effectiveness of NLP in handling unstructured data, such as free-text adverse event reports, demonstrates its potential to streamline pharmacovigilance processes. However, the accuracy and reliability of NLP algorithms must be rigorously validated. Organizations should invest in continuous improvement of these systems, incorporating feedback from pharmacovigilance professionals to enhance their performance. The potential of NLP to improve efficiency and accuracy in data processing makes it a valuable tool in the pharmacovigilance toolkit [75].

4.3 AI-driven signal detection

Signal detection is a critical component of pharmacovigilance, involving the identification of new safety signals from various data sources. A biotech company implemented an AI-driven signal detection system that analyzed data from clinical trials, post-marketing surveillance, social media, and scientific literature. The AI system used advanced algorithms to detect potential safety signals that might indicate new or emerging risks associated with their products.

4.3.1 Results

The AI-driven system proved to be highly effective, identifying several safety signals that had previously gone unnoticed [76]. This enabled the company to take timely action, such as updating product labels, issuing safety warnings, and conducting further investigations. The system's ability to analyze diverse data sources and detect signals in real-time significantly enhanced the company's pharmacovigilance capabilities.

4.3.2 Lessons learned

Integrating multiple data sources for comprehensive signal detection is crucial for a robust pharmacovigilance system. Ensuring the AI system is continuously monitored and validated is essential to maintain its effectiveness. Additionally, the AI-driven approach enhances the sensitivity and specificity of signal detection, allowing for earlier identification of potential risks and more proactive management of drug safety [77].

4.4 Patient engagement through AI-enabled platforms

Engaging patients in pharmacovigilance activities is crucial for collecting real-world data on drug safety. A healthcare organization developed an AI-enabled platform that allowed patients to report ADRs through a user-friendly mobile app. The platform used AI to analyze patient-reported data, providing real-time feedback and recommendations to patients and healthcare providers.

4.4.1 Results

The AI-enabled platform successfully increased patient participation in pharmacovigilance activities, leading to a richer dataset for drug safety analysis. Patients appreciated the convenience and responsiveness of the platform, while healthcare providers benefited from timely access to ADR information. The platform also facilitated better communication between patients and providers, improving overall patient care.

4.4.2 Lessons learned

The potential of AI-enabled platforms to enhance patient engagement in pharmacovigilance is significant. Designing user-friendly interfaces is key to encouraging patient participation. Real-time data analysis and feedback enhance the value of these platforms by providing timely insights that can improve drug safety monitoring and patient outcomes. The integration of patient-reported data adds a valuable dimension to pharmacovigilance, capturing insights that might otherwise be missed [78].

4.5 AI for post-marketing surveillance

Post-marketing surveillance is essential for monitoring the safety of drugs after they have been approved for use. A large pharmaceutical company implemented an AI system to analyze post-marketing data, including EHRs, social media, and adverse event reports. The AI system used machine learning algorithms to identify potential safety issues and trends in real-time.

4.5.1 Results

The implementation of the AI system led to several significant safety discoveries, prompting the company to take action to mitigate risks. For example, the AI system detected an increase in adverse events associated with a particular drug in a specific patient population. This information allowed the company to conduct further investigations and implement measures to ensure patient safety.

4.5.2 Lessons learned

AI plays a critical role in enhancing post-marketing surveillance by providing real-time analysis and early detection of safety issues. Comprehensive data integration and real-time analysis are necessary to identify emerging safety concerns effectively. Using AI to complement traditional pharmacovigilance methods enhances overall drug safety monitoring and provides a more complete picture of a drug's safety profile.

5. Implementation strategies

5.1 Technology selection

Choosing the right AI and ML technologies is the first step in implementing these tools in pharmacovigilance. Organizations must assess their specific needs and select technologies that align with their goals, considering factors such as data type, volume, and desired outcomes.

5.1.1 Pilot projects

Starting with pilot projects allows organizations to test AI and ML technologies on a smaller scale before full deployment [79]. These projects can help identify potential issues, refine algorithms, and demonstrate the value of AI-driven pharmacovigilance to stakeholders. Successful pilot projects should be designed to evaluate key performance metrics such as accuracy, speed, and scalability.

5.1.2 Vendor partnerships

Collaborating with technology vendors and AI experts can provide access to specialized knowledge and resources. Vendors can offer pre-built solutions tailored to pharmacovigilance needs, reducing the time and effort required for implementation. Additionally, vendor partnerships can provide ongoing support and updates, ensuring that AI systems remain cutting-edge.

5.2 Data quality management

Ensuring high-quality data is crucial for the success of AI and ML in pharmacovigilance. Data quality management involves several key activities, including data collection, cleaning, annotation, and integration.

5.2.1 Data collection

Effective data collection strategies ensure that the datasets used for training and analysis are comprehensive and representative. Organizations should establish standardized protocols for data collection, covering various sources such as clinical trials, electronic health records (EHRs), social media, and adverse event reports [80].

5.2.2 Data cleaning and annotation

Data cleaning involves removing errors, inconsistencies, and duplicates from datasets. This step is critical to prevent garbage-in, garbage-out scenarios where poor-quality data leads to inaccurate AI predictions. Data annotation, particularly for unstructured data, requires expert input to label data accurately. Techniques such as crowdsourcing and machine-assisted annotation can improve efficiency.

5.2.3 Data integration

Integrating data from multiple sources provides a holistic view of drug safety. Organizations should implement data integration frameworks that facilitate the seamless merging of structured and unstructured data. This may involve using data lakes, ETL (extract, transform, load) processes, and APIs (application programming interfaces) to ensure data compatibility and accessibility.

5.3 Workforce development

A skilled workforce is essential for the successful implementation of AI and ML in pharmacovigilance. Organizations must invest in training and development programs to equip their staff with the necessary skills and knowledge.

5.3.1 Training programs

Comprehensive training programs should cover the fundamentals of AI and ML, as well as their specific applications in pharmacovigilance. Topics may include data science, statistical analysis, programming languages (e.g., Python, R), and the use of AI tools and platforms. Continuous learning opportunities, such as workshops, webinars, and certifications, can help staff stay updated with the latest advancements [81].

5.3.2 Cross-disciplinary teams

Forming cross-disciplinary teams that combine expertise in pharmacovigilance, AI, data science, and regulatory affairs can enhance the implementation process. These teams can collaborate on developing, validating, and deploying AI models, ensuring that diverse perspectives and expertise are considered.

5.4 Regulatory compliance

Navigating the regulatory landscape is a critical component of AI and ML implementation in pharmacovigilance. Organizations must ensure that their AI-driven pharmacovigilance systems comply with regulatory requirements and ethical standards [82].

5.4.1 Engagement with regulators

Proactive engagement with regulatory bodies, such as the FDA and EMA, is essential for understanding and adhering to regulatory guidelines. Organizations should participate in regulatory consultations, provide feedback on draft regulations, and seek guidance on specific compliance issues.

5.4.2 Validation and monitoring

Regulatory compliance involves rigorous validation and continuous monitoring of AI systems. Validation ensures that AI models are accurate, reliable, and generalizable across different datasets. Post-deployment monitoring detects any deviations in model performance, enabling timely interventions and updates.

5.4.3 Ethical considerations

Adhering to ethical principles, such as data privacy, transparency, and fairness, is crucial for maintaining public trust. Organizations should implement robust data governance frameworks, conduct ethical audits, and ensure that AI systems are transparent and explainable.

5.5 Change management

Implementing AI and ML in pharmacovigilance requires effective change management to address organizational, cultural, and operational challenges.

5.5.1 Stakeholder engagement

Engaging stakeholders, including employees, regulators, patients, and healthcare providers, is essential for gaining buy-in and support. Clear communication of the benefits and implications of AI-driven pharmacovigilance can help address concerns and foster a positive attitude towards change [83].

5.5.2 Incremental implementation

Adopting an incremental approach to implementation allows organizations to manage change more effectively. By gradually scaling up AI and ML initiatives, organizations can minimize disruptions and build confidence in the new systems.

5.5.3 Performance metrics

Establishing clear performance metrics and key performance indicators (KPIs) helps track the success of AI and ML implementation. Metrics may include improvements in ADR detection rates, processing times, and overall efficiency. Regularly reviewing these metrics can inform continuous improvement efforts.

5.6 Conclusion

The integration of artificial intelligence (AI), machine learning (ML), and Big Data technologies into pharmacovigilance (PV) represents a transformative advancement in drug safety monitoring. As these technologies continue to evolve, their potential to enhance PV processes, predict adverse drug reactions (ADRs), and streamline data analysis becomes increasingly evident. This chapter has explored various facets of AI and ML in PV, highlighting their applications, challenges, and future directions.

5.7 Summary of key findings

Technological advances: AI and ML have revolutionized traditional PV methods, introducing capabilities such as predictive modeling, natural language processing (NLP), and real-time signal detection. These technologies enable more efficient and accurate identification of ADRs, improving the overall safety profile of medications.

Challenges: Despite the numerous benefits, the integration of AI and ML in PV is not without challenges. Ensuring data quality and consistency, navigating regulatory and compliance issues, managing technological integration, and addressing ethical considerations are critical hurdles that must be overcome. Organizations must adopt robust data governance frameworks, engage with regulatory bodies, and implement continuous monitoring and validation processes to address these challenges effectively.

Case studies: Real-world applications of AI and ML in PV demonstrate their potential to significantly enhance drug safety monitoring. Case studies on predictive modeling, NLP for adverse event reporting, AI-driven signal detection, patient engagement through AI-enabled platforms, and AI for post-marketing surveillance provide valuable insights into the practical implementation and impact of these technologies. For example, the application of deep learning models in pharmacovigilance has significantly enhanced the detection of ADRs by analyzing complex datasets more effectively than traditional statistical methods. These case studies illustrate the transformative potential of AI in improving drug safety monitoring and patient outcomes.

Implementation strategies: Successful implementation of AI and ML in PV requires strategic planning and execution. Key strategies include selecting appropriate technologies, ensuring data quality, fostering a skilled workforce, maintaining regulatory compliance, and managing organizational change. Pilot projects and vendor partnerships can facilitate initial implementation, while comprehensive training programs and cross-disciplinary teams are essential for long-term success.

5.8 Future directions

The future of PV lies in the continued advancement and integration of AI, ML, and Big Data technologies. Emerging trends such as advanced algorithms, predictive analytics, and real-time monitoring will further enhance PV capabilities. Additionally, the incorporation of ethical considerations, data privacy, and algorithmic fairness will be crucial for maintaining public trust and ensuring the responsible use of AI in healthcare.

Collaboration between stakeholders, including pharmaceutical companies, regulatory agencies, healthcare providers, and technology vendors, will be essential for the successful implementation and adoption of AI-driven PV systems. By working together, these stakeholders can develop harmonized regulations, share data and resources, and promote innovation in drug safety monitoring.

6. Conclusion

In conclusion, AI and ML hold immense promise for transforming PV, making it more proactive, efficient, and effective. By leveraging these technologies,

Data Source	Type of Data	Key Attributes	Examples
Clinical trials	Structured	Patient demographics, dosages, side effects	Phase I-III trial data
EHRs	Structured/unstructured	Diagnoses, treatment regimens, outcomes	Hospital records
Social media	Unstructured	Patient symptoms, experiences, sentiment	Twitter, patient forums

Table 8.
Summary of data sources and their characteristics.

organizations can enhance their ability to detect and manage ADRs, ultimately improving patient safety and public health. While challenges remain, the opportunities presented by AI and ML in PV are vast and far-reaching. As we continue to explore and refine these technologies, their impact on drug safety monitoring will undoubtedly grow, ushering in a new era of pharmacovigilance (**Table 8**).

7. Technological advances in pharmacovigilance

See (**Figure 1**).

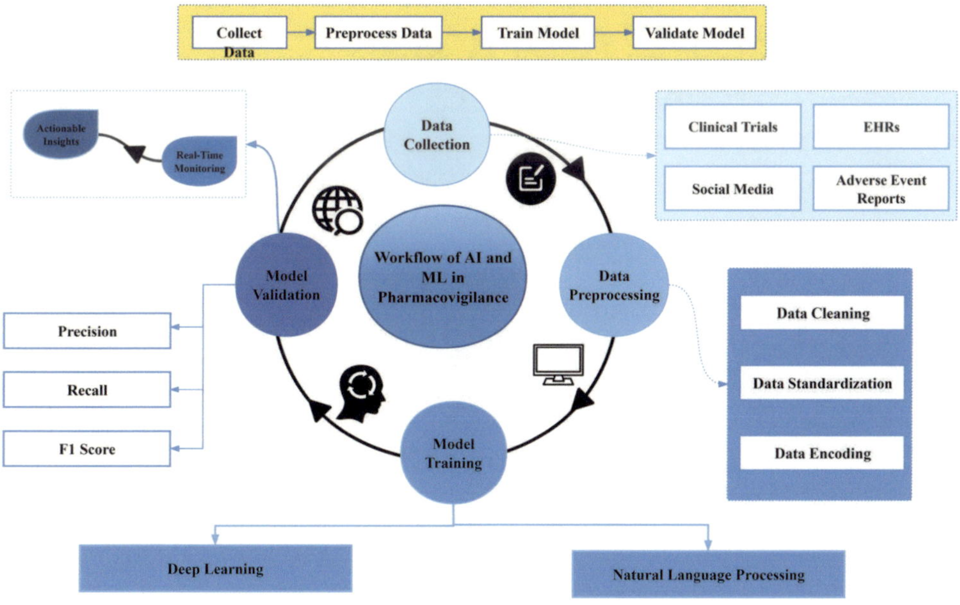

Figure 1.
Workflow of AI and ML in pharmacovigilance. Description: *This figure depicts the end-to-end workflow of implementing AI and ML in pharmacovigilance. The flowchart includes the following steps: 1.* Data collection: *Gathering data from various sources such as clinical trials, electronic health records (EHRs), social media, and adverse event reports. 2.* Data preprocessing: *Cleaning, standardizing, and encoding data to ensure quality and consistency. 3.* Model training: *Using historical data to train AI and ML models, including techniques like deep learning and natural language processing (NLP). 4.* Model validation: *Evaluating model performance using metrics such as precision, recall, and F1 score to ensure accuracy and reliability. 5.* Real-time monitoring: *Deploying models to analyze new data in real-time, identifying potential adverse drug reactions (ADRs) and safety signals. 6.* Actionable insights: *Generating reports and recommendations based on model outputs for healthcare providers and regulatory bodies to take necessary actions.*

8. Challenges and opportunities

See (**Table 9**).

Challenge	Description	Potential solutions
Data quality	Inconsistent and inaccurate data	Implement robust data governance, standardize data collection, continuous monitoring, and validation
Regulatory compliance	Evolving regulatory landscape and lack of clear guidelines	Engage proactively with regulators, participate in regulatory consultations, develop adaptive validation frameworks
Technological integration	Integration of diverse data sources and real-time processing	Invest in high-performance computing infrastructure, develop interoperability standards, and ensure seamless data integration
Ethical considerations	Data privacy, algorithmic bias, transparency, and accountability	Implement data encryption and anonymization, use fairness-aware ML techniques, adopt explainable AI (XAI) methods, establish clear accountability frameworks

Table 9.
Challenges and Solutions in Implementing AI in PV.

9. Case studies

See (**Figure 2** and **Table 10**).

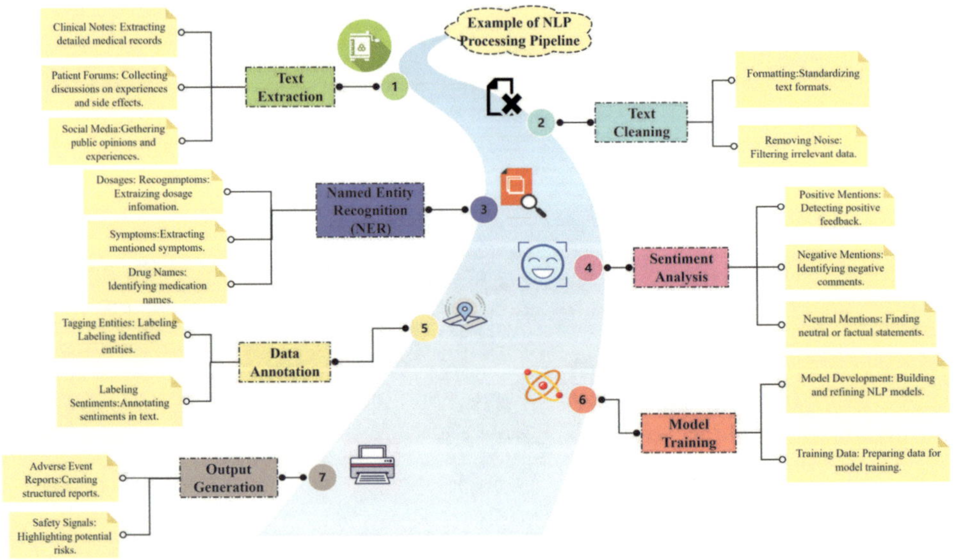

Figure 2.
Example of NLP Processing Pipeline. Description: *This figure illustrates the natural language processing (NLP) pipeline used for analyzing adverse event reports in pharmacovigilance. The diagram includes the following steps:* 1. Text extraction: *Collecting unstructured text data from sources such as clinical notes, patient forums, and social media.* 2. Text cleaning: *Removing noise, such as irrelevant information and formatting inconsistencies.* 3. Tokenization: *Breaking down text into individual words or phrases (tokens) for analysis.* 4. Named Entity Recognition (NER): *Identifying and classifying key entities such as drug names, symptoms, and dosages within the text.* 5. Sentiment Analysis: *Analyzing the sentiment expressed in the text to identify positive, negative, or neutral mentions of drugs and their effects.* 6. Data Annotation: *Labeling extracted information with relevant tags for further analysis.* 7. Model Training: *Using annotated data to train NLP models to recognize patterns and extract meaningful insights from new text data.* 8. Output Generation: *Producing structured data outputs, such as adverse event reports and safety signals, for further evaluation* (**Table 10**).

Model	Precision	Recall	F1 score	Novel ADRs identified
Deep learning A	0.92	0.88	0.90	Multiple, including rare conditions
NLP model B	0.89	0.85	0.87	Enhanced ADR detection from free-text data

Table 10.
Performance metrics of AI models for ADR detection.

10. Implementation strategies

See (**Figure 3**).
See (**Figure 4**).
See (**Figure 5**).
See (**Figure 6**).
See (**Figure 7**).
See (**Figure 8**).
See (**Figure 9**).

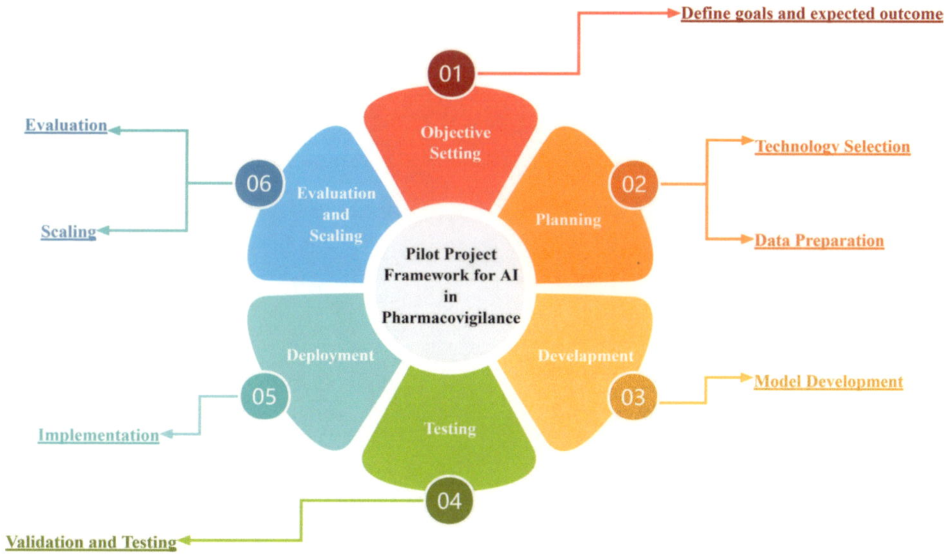

Figure 3.
Pilot Project Framework for AI in pharmacovigilance. Description: *This figure outlines the framework for conducting pilot projects to implement AI in pharmacovigilance. The framework includes the following components:* Objective setting: *Defining the goals and expected outcomes of the pilot project, such as improving ADR detection or streamlining adverse event reporting. 1.* Technology selection: *Choosing appropriate AI and ML technologies based on the project objectives and data requirements. 2.* Data preparation: *Collecting and preprocessing data from relevant sources, ensuring it is suitable for model training and analysis. 3.* Model development: *Building and training AI models using the prepared data, focusing on techniques such as deep learning and NLP. 4.* Validation and testing: *Evaluating model performance through rigorous testing and validation processes, using metrics like precision, recall, and F1 score. 5.* Implementation: *Deploying the validated models in a controlled environment to monitor their performance and gather initial results. 6.* Evaluation: *Assessing the outcomes of the pilot project against the defined objectives, identifying successes and areas for improvement. 7.* Scaling: *Based on the pilot project's success, planning the broader implementation of AI models in pharmacovigilance processes, including necessary adjustments and enhancements.*

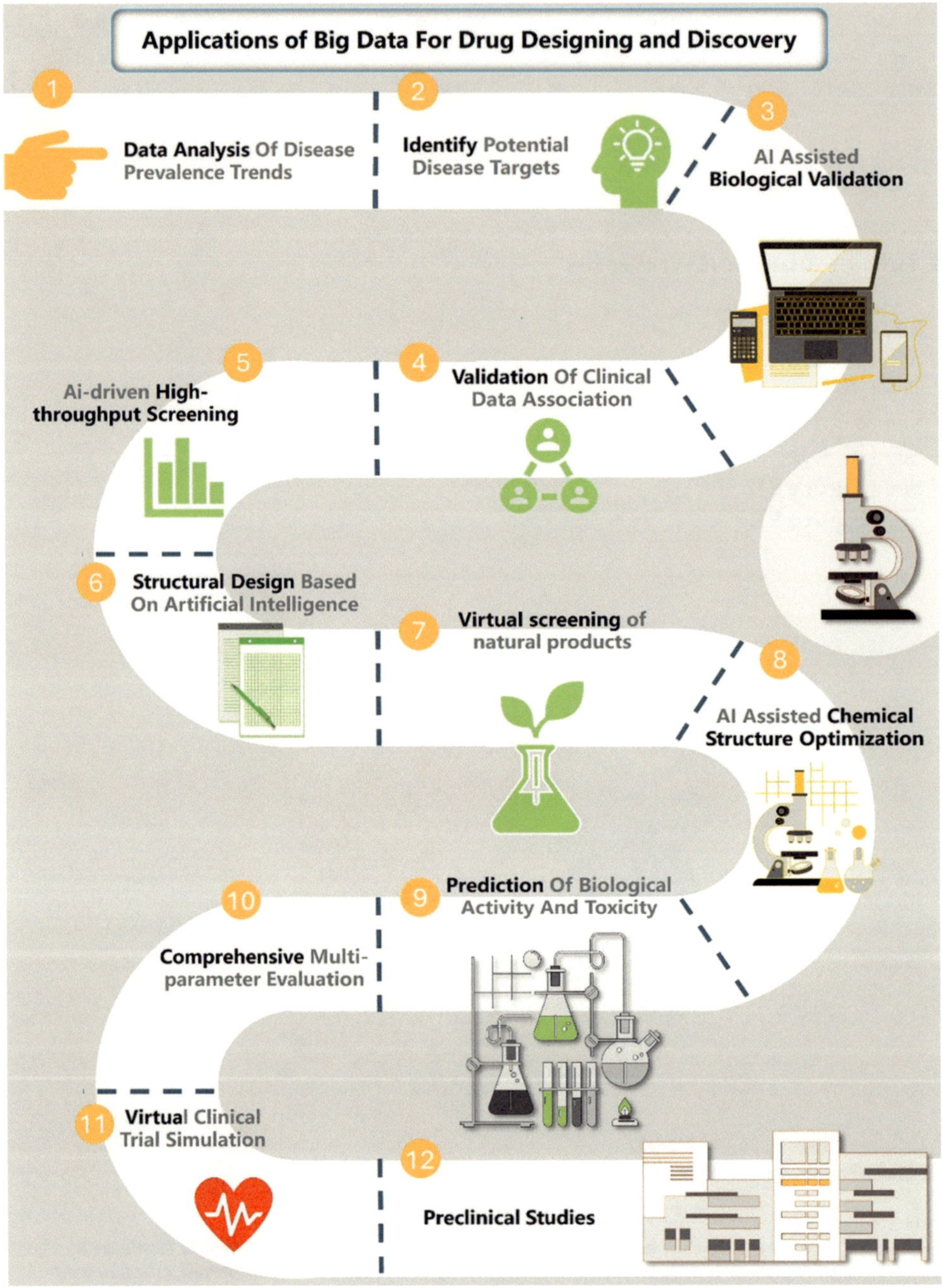

Figure 4.
Applications of big data for drug designing and discovery. Note: *This graphic illustrates how artificial intelligence (AI) is transforming drug design and discovery by addressing major challenges such as long development timelines, high costs, and inefficiencies. It showcases the application of AI algorithms, including machine learning and deep learning, in critical areas like molecular design, virtual screening, molecular docking, and toxicity prediction. This highlights AI's role in enhancing precision, speed, and innovation across the entire drug development process.*

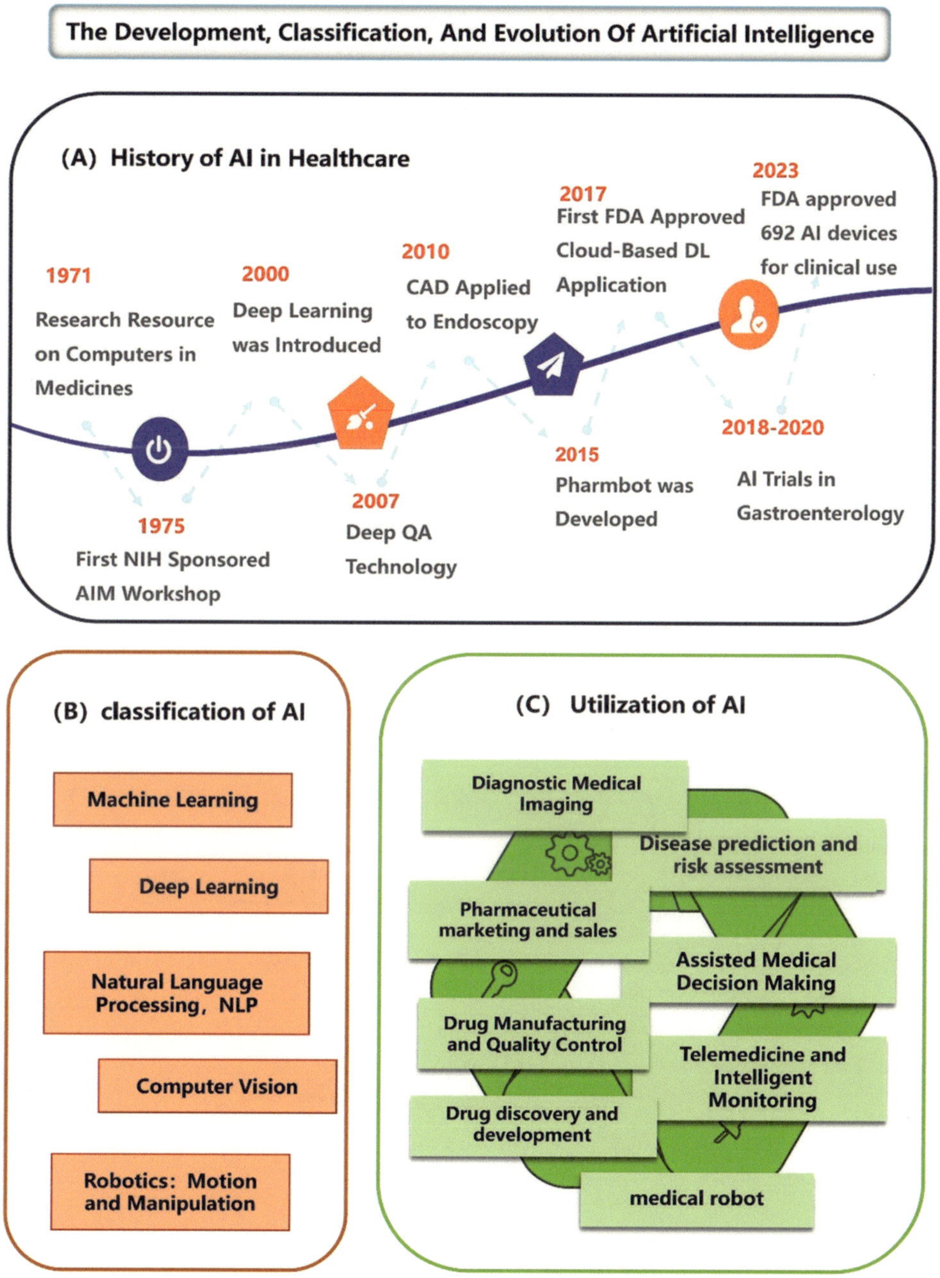

Figure 5.
The development, classification, and evolution of artificial intelligence. a. History: *AI in healthcare began with the 1950 Turing test, followed by milestones like the 1975 use of computers in medicine, deep learning in the 2000s, and FDA's approval of the first cloud-based AI in 2017. Key developments include AI in endoscopy (2010) and gastroenterology trials (2018–2020).* b. Classification: *AI divides into seven areas: reasoning, knowledge representation, planning, perception, machine learning, robotics, and NLP. Machine learning includes supervised, unsupervised, and deep learning; vision and speech cover image recognition and speech-to-text; NLP includes classification, translation, and question answering.* c. Applications in Healthcare: *AI's impact spans research, clinical development, manufacturing, patient monitoring, and post-market surveillance, transforming healthcare.*

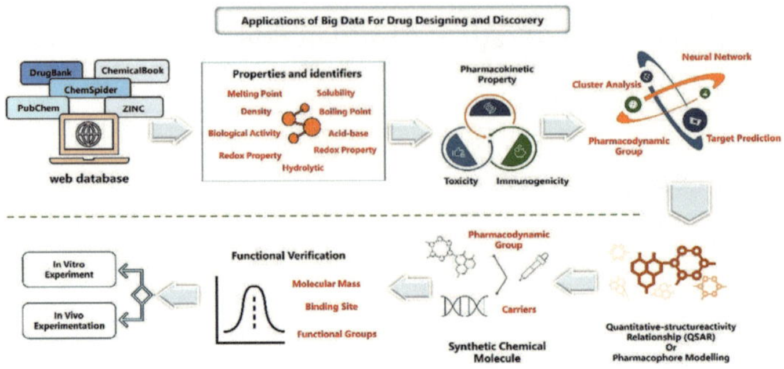

Figure 6.
Applications of big data for drug designing and discovery. Note: *This figure illustrates how big data supports drug design and discovery by utilizing key databases like ChemSpider, ChEMBL, ZINC, BindingDB, and PubChem, which compile pharmacological data to aid compound synthesis and screening. Following initial filters for drug-likeness, PAINS, ADMET, and toxicity, AI models such as deep learning and random forest conduct in-depth compound analysis. The workflow advances with QSAR, pharmacophore modeling, molecular docking, and dynamics simulations, ultimately identifying candidate compounds for in vitro and in vivo testing. Quantum mechanics contributes to this process, with its role in drug design continuously evolving.*

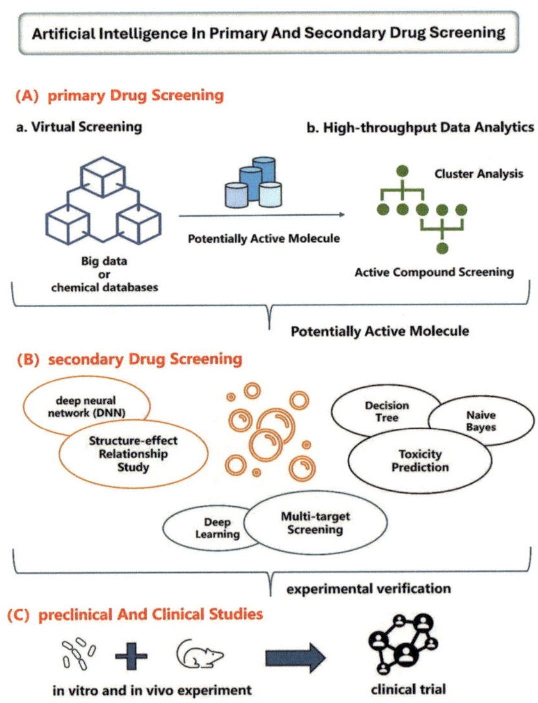

Figure 7.
Artificial intelligence in primary and secondary drug screening. Note: *This figure illustrates how AI expedites drug screening by identifying lead compounds from a vast chemical space of over 106 million structures. Machine learning models help screen these compounds for target binding and structural properties. This AI-driven drug discovery process, typically spanning 14–18 years, encompasses lead identification, primary and secondary screening, lead optimization, and clinical development.*

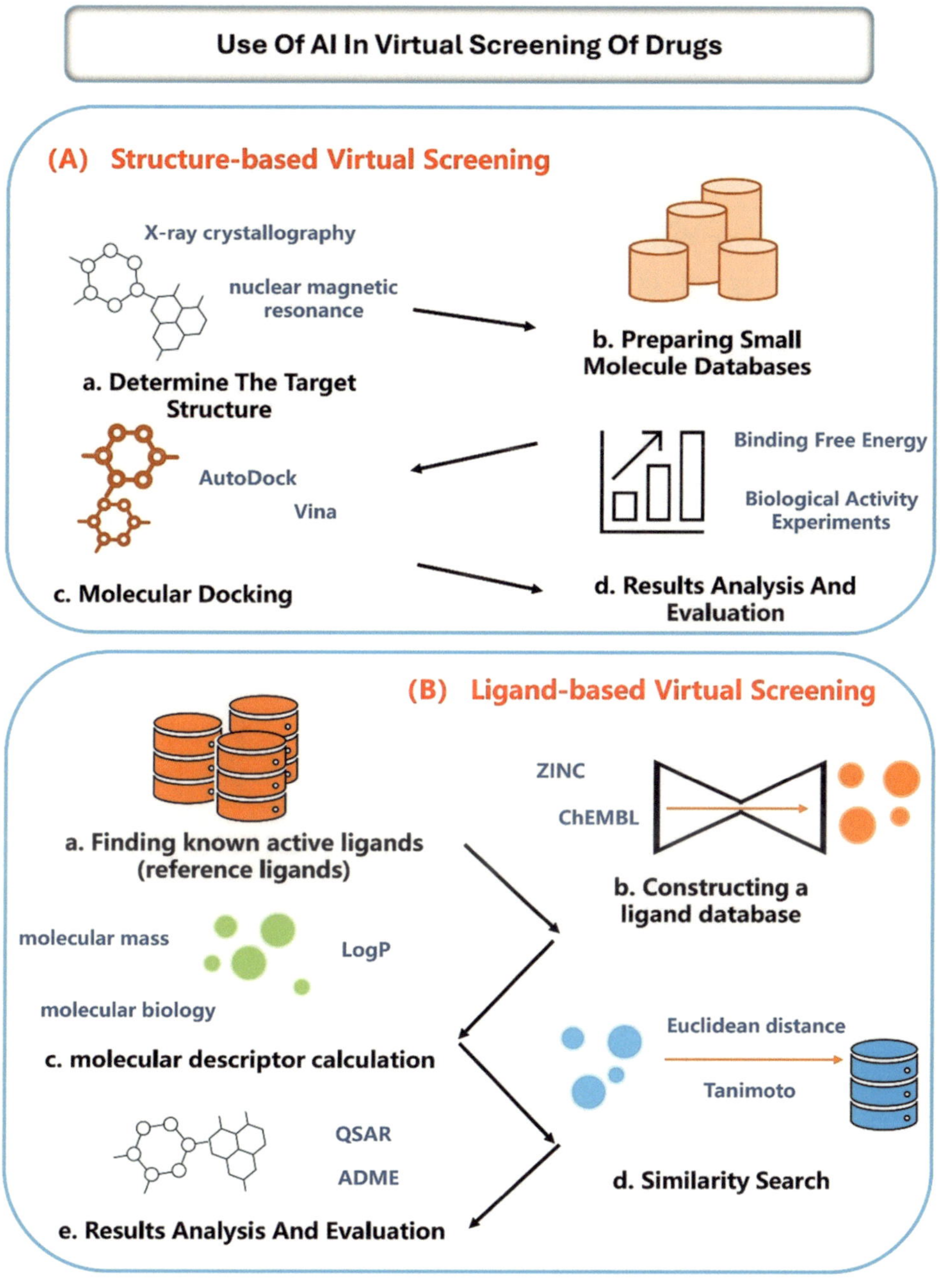

Figure 8.
Use of AI in virtual screening of drugs. Note: *This figure highlights two primary virtual screening methods in drug discovery: a.* Structure-based virtual screening: *This approach involves preparing the target and chemical library, analyzing structural features, predicting binding sites, and conducting molecular docking. Screened compounds are then validated with molecular dynamics simulations and confirmed through experimental bioassays. b.* Ligand-based virtual screening: *This method starts with database screening and 3D structural modeling of targets, followed by pharmacophore modeling and docking-based screening. Screened compounds undergo toxicity and physicochemical analysis before final validation via in vitro and in vivo bioassays.*

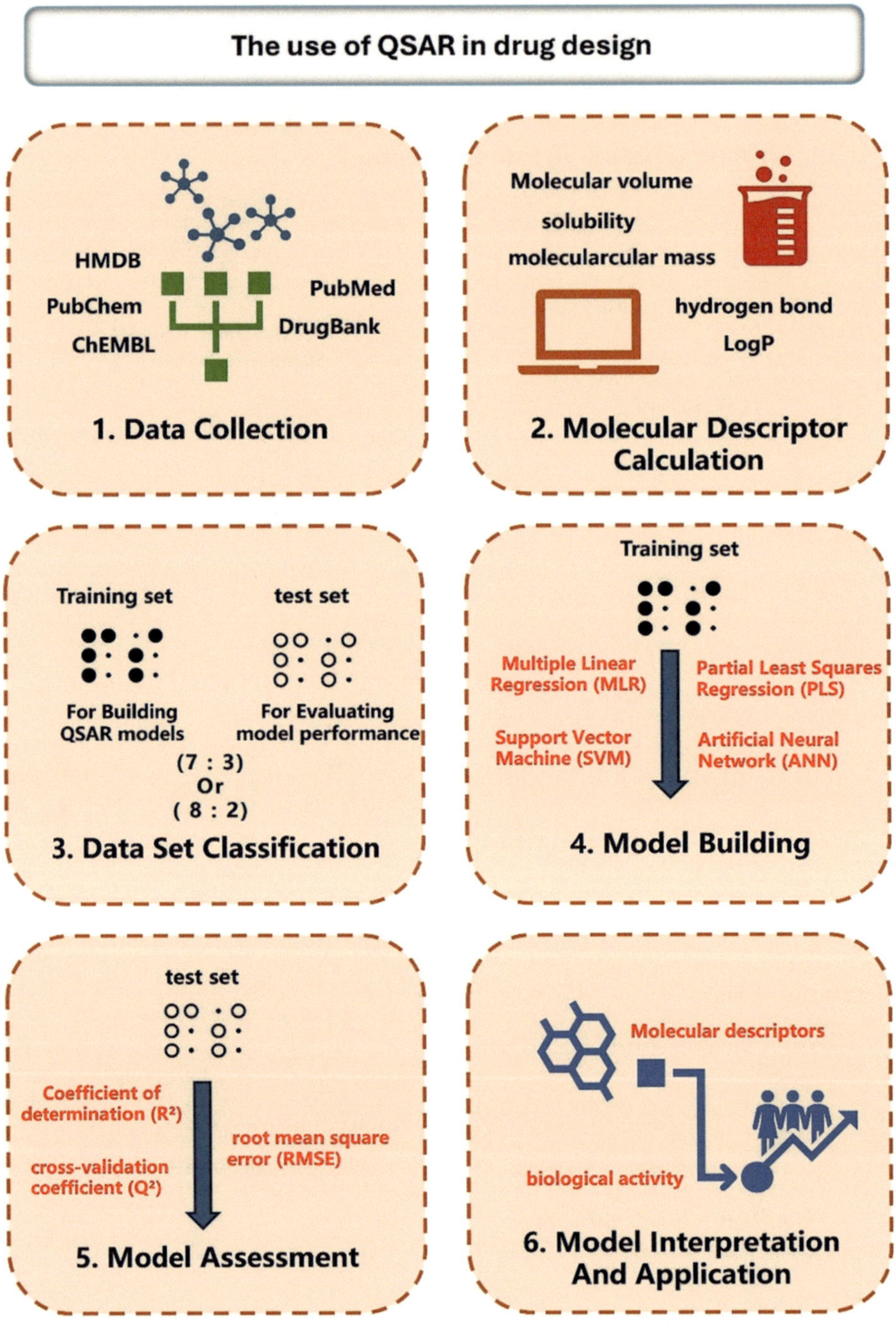

Figure 9.
The use of QSAR in drug design. Note: *This figure highlights essential workflows in drug discovery: a.* QSAR workflow: *Begins with data compilation and processing, involving descriptor calculation and dataset splitting. Model construction employs machine learning algorithms, followed by robustness assessment and benchmarking. b.* Drug repurposing workflow: *Starts with data collection and model generation using methods like support vector machines and deep learning. The workflow concludes with model evaluation and validation through clinical trials and experimental studies.*

Author details

Jian Yang[1,2,3,4] and Fan Li[1,2,3,4*]

1 School of Pharmaceutical Sciences and Yunnan Provincial Key Laboratory of Pharmacology for Natural Products, Kunming Medical University, Kunming, Yunnan, China

2 Yunnan Provincial Center for Drug Policy Research, Kunming, Yunnan, China

3 College of Modern Biomedical Industry, Kunming Medical University, Kunming, Yunnan, China

4 Technology Transfer Center, Kunming Medical University, Kunming, Yunnan, China

*Address all correspondence to: 1425256831@qq.com

IntechOpen

© 2024 The Author(s). Licensee IntechOpen. This chapter is distributed under the terms of the Creative Commons Attribution License (http://creativecommons.org/licenses/by/4.0), which permits unrestricted use, distribution, and reproduction in any medium, provided the original work is properly cited.

References

[1] Abatemarco D, Perera S, Bao SH, Desai S, Assuncao B, Tetarenko N, et al. Training augmented intelligent capabilities for pharmacovigilance: Applying deep-learning approaches to individual case safety report processing. Pharmaceutical Medicine. 2018;**32**(6):391-401

[2] Standing Committee of the National People's Congress. Medicinal Product Administration Law of the People's Republic of China. 2019. Revision. Available from: http://www.gov.cn/banshi/2005-08/01/content_18993.htm [Accessed: October 2, 2021]

[3] Fornasier G, Francescon S, Leone R, Baldo P. An historical overview over pharmacovigilance. International Journal of Clinical Pharmacology. 2018;**40**(4):744-747. DOI: 10.1007/s11096-018-0657-1

[4] Bates DW, Levine D, Syrowatka A, Kuznetsova M, Craig KJT, Rui A, et al. The potential of artificial intelligence to improve patient safety: A scoping review. npj Digital Medicine. 2021;**4**(1):54

[5] Macrae C. Governing the safety of artificial intelligence in healthcare. BMJ Quality and Safety. 2019;**28**(6):495-498

[6] Jiao XF, Li HL, Jiao XY, et al. Ovary and uterus related adverse events associated with statin use: An analysis of the FDA adverse event reporting system. Scientific Reports. 2020;**10**:1-10. DOI: 10.1038/s41598-020-68906-2

[7] Colacci M, Fralick M. Have current systems of pharmacovigilance had their day?: The "pro" side. The Canadian Journal of Hospital Pharmacy. 2020;**73**(2):159-160. DOI: 10.4212/cjhp.v73i2.3186

[8] Basile AO, Yahi A, Tatonetti NP. Artificial intelligence for drug toxicity and safety. Trends in Pharmacological Sciences. 2019;**40**(9):624-635

[9] Ben Abacha A, Chowdhury MFM, Karanasiou A, Mrabet Y, Lavelli A, Zweigenbaum P. Text mining for pharmacovigilance: Using machine learning for drug name recognition and drug-drug interaction extraction and classification. Journal of Biomedical Informatics. 2015;**58**:122-132

[10] Chandak P, Tatonetti NP. Using machine learning to identify adverse drug effects posing increased risk to women. Patterns (NY). 2020;**1**(7):100108

[11] Calix RA, Gupta R, Gupta M, Jiang K, editors. Deep granulator: Improving precision in the classification of personal health-experience tweets with deep learning. In: 2017 IEEE International Conference on Bioinformatics and Biomedicine (BIBM). Kansas City, MO, USA: IEEE Computer Society; 2017. pp. 1154-1159

[12] Benin AL, Fodeh SJ, Lee K, Koss M, Miller P, Brandt C. Electronic approaches to making sense of the text in the adverse event reporting system. Journal of Healthcare Risk Management. 2016;**36**(2):10-20

[13] Chen Z, Zhang H, George T, Prosperi M, Guo Y, Braithwaite D, et al. Abstract PO-071: Simulation of colorectal cancer clinical trials using real-world data and machine learning. Clinical Cancer Research. 2021;**27**(Suppl. 5):PO-071

[14] Das S, Dey A, Pal A, Roy N. Applications of artificial intelligence in machine learning: Review and prospect. International Journal of Computers and Applications. 2015;**115**:31-41

[15] Hashimoto DA, Rosman G, Rus D, Meireles OR. Artificial intelligence in surgery: Promises and perils. Annals of Surgery. 2018;**268**(1):70-76

[16] Bouzillé G, Morival C, Westerlynck R, Lemordant P, Chazard E, Lecorre P, et al. An automated detection system of drug-drug interactions from electronic patient records using big data analytics. Studies in Health Technology and Informatics. 2019;**264**:45-49

[17] WHO. The importance of pharmacovigilance. Available from: https://apps.who.int/iris/bitstream/handle/10665/42493/a75646.pdf [Accessed: October 2, 2021]

[18] Cocos A, Fiks AG, Masino AJ. Deep learning for pharmacovigilance: Recurrent neural network architectures for labeling adverse drug reactions in twitter posts. Journal of the American Medical Informatics Association. 2017;**24**(4):813-821

[19] Colón-Ruiz C, Segura-Bedmar I. Comparing deep learning architectures for sentiment analysis on drug reviews. Journal of Biomedical Informatics. 2020;**110**:103539

[20] Comfort S, Perera S, Hudson Z, Dorrell D, Meireis S, Nagarajan M, et al. Sorting through the safety data haystack: Using machine learning to identify individual case safety reports in social-digital media. Drug Safety. 2018;**41**(6):579-590

[21] Dandala B, Joopudi V, Devarakonda M. Adverse drug events detection in clinical notes by jointly modeling entities and relations using neural networks. Drug Safety. 2019;**42**(1):135-146

[22] Correia Pinheiro L, Durand J, Dogné JM. An application of machine learning in pharmacovigilance: Estimating likely patient genotype from phenotypical manifestations of fluoropyrimidine toxicity. Clinical Pharmacology and Therapeutics. 2020;**107**(4):944-947

[23] De Pretis F, Landes J, Peden W. Artificial intelligence methods for a Bayesian epistemology-powered evidence evaluation. Journal of Evaluation in Clinical Practice. 2021;**27**(3):504-512

[24] Desai S, Chan K, Bannout K, Mingle E, Freeman J, Parikh U, et al. A novel approach to standardizing data and detecting duplicates across adverse event data sources using machine learning. Drug Safety. 2018;**41**(11):1246-1247

[25] El-Allaly ED, Sarrouti M, En-Nahnahi N, Ouatik El Alaoui S. An adverse drug effect mentions extraction method based on weighted online recurrent extreme learning machine. Computer Methods and Programs in Biomedicine. 2019;**176**:33-41

[26] Desai SME, Egan B, Gulati R, Freeman J. A framework for leveraging emerging technologies in pharmacovigilance. Drug Safety. 2018;**41**(11):1223-1224

[27] Evans HP, Anastasiou A, Edwards A, Hibbert P, Makeham M, Luz S, et al. Automated classification of primary care patient safety incident report content and severity using supervised machine learning (ML) approaches. Health Informatics Journal. 2019;**26**(4):3123-3139

[28] Davazdahemami B, Delen D. A chronological pharmacovigilance network analytics approach for predicting adverse drug events. Journal of the American Medical Informatics Association. 2018;**25**(10):1311-1321

[29] Fan Y, Zhang R. Using natural language processing methods to classify use status of dietary supplements in clinical notes. BMC Medical Informatics and Decision Making. 2018;**18**(2):51

[30] Fan Y, He L, Zhang R. Evaluating automatic methods to extract patients' supplement use from clinical reports. Proceedings IEEE International Conference on Bioinformatics and Biomedicine. 2017;**2017**:1258-1261

[31] Hazell L, Shakir SA. Under-reporting of adverse drug reactis: A systematic review. Drug Safety. 2006;**29**(5):385-396. DOI: 10.2165/00002018-200629050-00003

[32] Fong A, Harriott N, Walters DM, Foley H, Morrissey R, Ratwani RR. Integrating natural language processing expertise with patient safety event review committees to improve the analysis of medication events. International Journal of Medical Informatics. 2017;**104**:120-125

[33] Fong A, Behzad S, Pruitt Z, Ratwani RM. A machine learning approach to reclassifying miscellaneous patient safety event reports. Journal of Patient Safety. 2021;**17**(8):33

[34] Fernandez-Fernandez C, Lázaro-Bengoa E, Fernández-Antón E, Quiroga-González L, Montero CD. Quantity is not enough: Completeness of suspected adverse drug reaction reports in Spain – Differences between regional pharmacovigilance centres and pharmaceutical industry. European Journal of Clinical Pharmacology. 2020;**76**(8):1175-1181. DOI: 10.1007/s00228-020-02894-0

[35] Gartland A, Bate A, Painter JL, Casperson TA, Powell GE. Developing crowdsourced training data sets for pharmacovigilance intelligent automation. Drug Safety. 2021;**44**(3):373-382

[36] Gupta S, Pawar S, Ramrakhiyani N, Palshikar GK, Varma V. Semi-supervised recurrent neural network for adverse drug reaction mention extraction. BMC Bioinformatics. 2018;**19**(8):212

[37] Foufi V, Ing Lorenzini K, Goldman JP, Gaudet-Blavignac C, Lovis C, Samer C. Automatic classification of discharge letters to detect adverse drug reactions. Studies in Health Technology and Informatics. 2020;**270**:48-52

[38] Kreimeyer K, Dang O, Spiker J, Muñoz MA, Rosner G, Ball R, et al. Feature engineering and machine learning for causality assessment in pharmacovigilance: Lessons learned from application to the FDA adverse event reporting system. Computers in Biology and Medicine. 2021;**135**:104517

[39] Laves M-H, Ihler S, Ortmaier T, Kahrs LA. Quantifying the uncertainty of deep learning-based computer-aided diagnosis for patient safety. Current Directions in Biomedical Engineering. 2019;**5**:223-226

[40] Letinier LJJ, Miremont G, Bel-Letoile A, Salvo F, Rouby F, et al. Machine learning and semantic information for unstructured healthcare data: Comparison of methods through the automatic analysis of adverse drug reaction reports. MAI TAI study. Fundam Clin Pharmacol. 2021;**35**(Suppl. 1):20

[41] Marella WM, Sparnon E, Finley E. Screening electronic health record-related patient safety reports using machine learning. Journal of Patient Safety. 2017;**13**(1):31-36

[42] Li F, Liu W, Yu H. Extraction of information related to adverse drug

events from electronic health record notes: Design of an end-to-end model based on deep learning. JMIR Medical Informatics. 2018;**6**(4):e12159

[43] Mockute R, Desai S, Perera S, Assuncao B, Danysz K, Tetarenko N, et al. Artificial intelligence within pharmacovigilance: A means to identify cognitive services and the framework for their validation. Pharmaceut Med. 2019;**33**(2):109-120

[44] Mower J, Subramanian D, Cohen T. Learning predictive models of drug side-effect relationships from distributed representations of literature-derived semantic predications. Journal of the American Medical Informatics Association. 2018;**25**(10):1339-1350

[45] Negi K, Pavuri A, Patel L, Jain C. A novel method for drug-adverse event extraction using machine learning. Informatics in Medicine Unlocked. 2019;**17**:100190

[46] Schmider J, Kumar K, LaForest C, Swankoski B, Naim K, Caubel PM. Innovation in pharmacovigilance: Use of artificial intelligence in adverse event case processing. Clinical Pharmacology and Therapeutics. 2019;**105**(4):954-961

[47] Goldman A, Bomze D, Dankner R, et al. Cardiovascular adverse events associated with hydroxychloroquine and chloroquine: A comprehensive pharmacovigilance analysis of pre-COVID-19 reports. British Journal of Clinical Pharmacology. 2021;**87**(3):1432-1442. DOI: 10.1111/bcp.14546

[48] Yang J, Wang L, Phadke NA, Wickner PG, Mancini CM, Blumenthal KG, et al. Development and validation of a deep learning model for detection of allergic reactions using safety event reports across hospitals. JAMA Netw Open. 2 Nov 2020;**3**(11):e2022836

[49] Bond CM. Have current systems of pharmacovigilance had their day?: The "con" side. The Canadian Journal of Hospital Pharmacy. 2020;**73**:160-162. DOI: 10.4212/cjhp.v73i2.2983

[50] Yang X, Bian J, Gong Y, Hogan WR, Wu Y. MADEx: A system for detecting medications, adverse drug events, and their relations from clinical notes. Drug Safety. 2019;**42**(1):123-133

[51] Simon ST, Mandair D, Tiwari P, Rosenberg MA. Prediction of drug-induced long QT syndrome using machine learning applied to harmonized electronic health record data. Journal of Cardiovascular Pharmacology and Therapeutics. 2021;**26**(4):335-340

[52] Noguchi Y, Tachi T, Teramachi H. Subset analysis for screening drug-drug interaction signal using pharmacovigilance database. Pharmaceutics. 2020;**12**(8):762

[53] Létinier L, Jouganous J, Benkebil M, Bel-Létoile A, Goehrs C, Singier A, et al. Artificial intelligence for unstructured healthcare data: Application to coding of patient reporting of adverse drug reactions. Clinical Pharmacology and Therapeutics. 2021;**110**(2):392-400. DOI: 10.1002/cpt.2266

[54] Martin GL, Jouganous J, Savidan R, Bellec A, Goehrs C, Benkebil M, et al. Validation of artificial intelligence to support the automatic coding of patient adverse drug reaction reports, using nationwide pharmacovigilance data. Drug Safety. 2022;**45**(5):535-548. DOI: 10.1007/s40264-022-01153-8

[55] Routray R, Tetarenko N, Abu-Assal C, Mockute R, Assuncao B, Chen H, et al. Application of augmented intelligence for pharmacovigilance case seriousness determination. Drug Safety. 2020;**43**(1):57-66. DOI: 10.1007/s40264-019-00869-4

[56] Luo Y, Thompson WK, Herr TM, Zeng Z, Berendsen MA, Jonnalagadda SR, et al. Natural language processing for EHR-based pharmacovigilance: A structured review. Drug Safety. 2017;**40**(11):1075-1089. DOI: 10.1007/s40264-017-0558-6

[57] Murali K, Kaur S, Prakash A, Medhi B. Artificial intelligence in pharmacovigilance: Practical utility. Indian Journal Of Pharmacology. 2019;**51**(6):373. DOI: 10.4103/ijp.IJP_814_19

[58] Hauben M, Hartford CG. Artificial intelligence in pharmacovigilance: Scoping points to consider. Clinical Therapeutics. 2021;**43**(2):372-379. DOI: 10.1016/j.clinthera.2020.12.014

[59] Sarker A, Belousov M, Friedrichs J, Hakala K, Kiritchenko S, Mehryary F, et al. Data and systems for medication-related text classification and concept normalization from twitter: Insights from the social media mining for health (SMM4H)-2017 shared task. Journal of the American Medical Informatics Association. 2018;**25**(10):1274-1283. DOI: 10.1093/jamia/ocy114

[60] Niazi SK. The coming of age of AI/ML in drug discovery, development, clinical testing, and manufacturing: The FDA perspectives. Drug Design, Development and Therapy. 2023;**17**:2691-2725. DOI: 10.2147/DDDT.S424991

[61] Suriyaamporn P, Pamornpathomkul B, Patrojanasophon P, Ngawhirunpat T, Rojanarata T, Opanasopit P. The artificial intelligence-powered new era in pharmaceutical Research and Development: A review. AAPS PharmSciTech. 2024;**25**(6):188. DOI: 10.1208/s12249-024-02901-y

[62] Shiammala PN, Duraimutharasan NKB, Vaseeharan B, Alothaim AS, Al-Malki ES, Snekaa B, et al. Exploring the artificial intelligence and machine learning models in the context of drug design difficulties and future potential for the pharmaceutical sectors. Methods. 2023;**219**:82-94. DOI: 10.1016/j.ymeth.2023.09.010. Epub 2023 Sep 29

[63] Gupta R, Srivastava D, Sahu M, Tiwari S, Ambasta RK, Kumar P. Artificial intelligence to deep learning: Machine intelligence approach for drug discovery. Molecular Diversity. 2021;**25**(3):1315-1360. DOI: 10.1007/s11030-021-10217-3

[64] Hamet P, Tremblay J. Artificial intelligence in medicine. Metabolism. 2017;**69**:S36-S40. DOI: 10.1016/j.metabol.2017.01.011

[65] Hassanzadeh P, Atyabi F, Dinarvand R. The significance of artificial intelligence in drug delivery system design. Advanced Drug Delivery Reviews. 2019;**144**:103-115. DOI: 10.1016/j.addr.2019.05.001

[66] Zhang L, Tan J, Han D, Zhu H. From machine learning to deep learning: Progress in machine intelligence for rational drug discovery. Drug Discovery Today. 2017;**22**(11):1680-1685. DOI: 10.1016/j.drudis.2017.08.010

[67] Jordan AM. Artificial intelligence in drug design–the storm before the calm? ACS Medicinal Chemistry Letters. 2018;**9**(2):121-123. DOI: 10.1021/acsmedchemlett.8b00500

[68] Harrer S, Shah P, Antony B, Hu J. Artificial intelligence for clinical trial design. Trends in Pharmacological Sciences (TIPS). 2019;**40**(2):107-118

[69] Badillo S, Banfai B, Birzele F, et al. An introduction to machine learning. Clinical Pharmacology and Therapeutics. 2020;**107**(3):590-600. DOI: 10.1002/cpt.1796

[70] Schmidhuber J. Deep learning in neural networks: An overview. Neural Networks. 2015;**61**:85-117. DOI: 10.1016/j.neunet.2014.09.003

[71] Ilievski A, Zdraveski V, Gusev M. How CUDA powers the machine learning revolution. In: 2018 26th Telecommunications Forum (TELFOR). Belgrade, Serbia; 2018. pp. 420-425. DOI: 10.1109/TELFOR.2018.8611982

[72] Gandomi A, Haider M. Beyond the hype: Big data concepts, methods, and analytics. International Journal of Information Management. 2015;**35**:137-144. DOI: 10.1016/j.ijinfomgt.2014.10.007

[73] Han Y, Yang J, Qian X, et al. DriverML: A machine learning algorithm for identifying driver genes in cancer sequencing studies. Nucleic Acids Research. 2019;**47**(3):e19-e19. DOI: 10.1093/nar/gkz096

[74] Fan Y, Zhang Y, Hua Y, et al. Investigation of machine intelligence in compound cell activity classification. Molecular Pharmaceutics. 2019;**16**(10):4530-4538. DOI: 10.1021/acs.molpharmaceut.9b00558

[75] Jing Y, Bian Y, Hu Z, et al. Deep learning for drug design: An artificial intelligence paradigm for drug discovery in the big data era. The AAPS Journal. 2018;**20**(3):58. DOI: 10.1208/s12248-018-0210-0

[76] Gastegger M, McSloy A, Luya M, et al. A deep neural network for molecular wave functions in quasi-atomic minimal basis representation. The Journal of Chemical Physics. 2020;**153**(14):144111. DOI: 10.1063/5.0012911

[77] Davenport TH, Ronanki R. Artificial intelligence for the real world. Harvard Business Review. 2018;**96**(1):108-116

[78] Zhavoronkov A, Vanhaelen Q, Oprea TI. Will artificial intelligence for drug discovery impact clinical pharmacology? Clinical Pharmacology and Therapeutics. 2020;**107**(4):754-757. DOI: 10.1002/cpt.1795

[79] Elton DC, Boukouvalas Z, Butrico MS, et al. Applying machine learning techniques to predict the properties of energetic materials. Scientific Reports. 2018;**8**:9059. DOI: 10.1038/s41598-018-27344-x

[80] Zheng MJ, Cheng R, Song HB. Bibliometric analysis of pharmacovigilance research in China. Chinese Journal of Pharmacovigilance. 2021;**18**:686-688+696

[81] Embi PJ. Algorithmovigilance – Advancing methods to analyze and monitor artificial intelligence-driven health care for effectiveness and equity. JAMA Network Open. 2021;**4**(4):e214622. DOI: 10.1001/jamanetworkopen.2021.4622

[82] ICMRA. Horizon scanning assessment report – Artificial intelligence. Available from: http://www.icmra.info/drupal/sites/default/files/2021-08/horizon_scanning_report_artificial_intelligence.pdf [Accessed: October 2, 2021]

[83] Zou M, Barmaz Y, Preovolos M, Popko L, Ménard T. Using statistical modeling for enhanced and flexible pharmacovigilance audit risk assessment and planning. Therapeutic Innovation & Regulatory Science. 2021;**55**(1):190-196. DOI: 10.1007/s43441-020-00205-4

Section 2

Perspective Chapters: Challenges and Proposed Solutions in Different Countries

Chapter 4

Perspective Chapter: Challenges and Possible Solutions of ADR Monitoring (Pharmacovigilance) in Low- and Middle-Income Countries

Anant Khot and Ganesh Dakhale

Abstract

Pharmacovigilance (PV) is a crucial player in ensuring patient safety. It monitors and evaluates the safety of medicines, particularly in addressing adverse drug reactions (ADRs). However, low- and middle-income countries (LMICs) face unique challenges in establishing robust PV systems. Even in jurisdictions where reporting is mandatory, the underreporting of ADRs remains significant. The scarcity of professionals with expertise in PV, limited funding, and lack of public engagement further hinder the effectiveness of PV programmes. Inaccessibility to reporting forms, language barriers, and the complexity of the healthcare system also contribute to the challenges. Regulation-related issues, such as insufficient legislation and weak accountability of the pharmaceutical industry, pose additional obstacles. Healthcare professionals may refrain from reporting ADRs due to fear of professional dignity attrition and the absence of explicit legal provisions ensuring confidentiality. Clinical trials have limitations in detecting rare events, and attitudes towards ADR reporting, such as lack of time and incentives, further complicate the situation. Despite these challenges, establishing robust PV systems in LMICs can generate valuable data to inform crucial healthcare policy and practice decisions, potentially leading to significant improvements in patient safety and care.

Keywords: pharmacovigilance, adverse drug reactions, low- and middle-income countries, underreporting, patient safety

1. Introduction

The process of monitoring and evaluating the safety of medicines, known as pharmacovigilance (PV), is a critical component of healthcare. It focuses on detecting drug-related adverse reactions (ADRs) and any unintended and harmful effects of medications to ensure patient safety [1]. Studies indicate that ADRs are the sixth leading cause of death globally, resulting in nearly 7% of hospitalisations for patients [2]. In low-resource countries, the complex and fragmented nature of the healthcare system

IntechOpen

presents unique challenges that require immediate attention [3]. The pharmaceutical supply chain, comprised of entities, individuals, processes, and resources involved in delivering drugs from manufacturers to patients, is often hindered by weak regulatory supervision and poor enforcement of laws [4]. This vulnerability allows for the infiltration of substandard/spurious/falsely labelled/falsified/counterfeit (SSFFC) medicines and vaccines, leading to ADRs. In this context, PV activities play a crucial role as the first line of defence in identifying rare but potentially harmful ADRs, including those that emerge after prolonged exposure and drug-drug and drug-disease interactions that may not have been captured in randomised trials conducted before a drug's licencing [5]. However, the underreporting of ADRs remains a significant issue, even in jurisdictions where reporting is mandatory. The global data on ADRs, primarily from Western industrialised countries, are essential for assessing drug safety in other nations. However, these data may not always be applicable or suitable for specific settings or population groups due to genetic, physiological, cultural, environmental, and socio-behavioural differences among populations, which can significantly influence a population's response to certain medications. This complex and urgent topic is the focus of our discussion [6]. Low- and middle-income countries (LMICs) face unique challenges in establishing robust pharmacovigilance systems. However, when in place, these systems can generate data that inform crucial healthcare policy and practice decisions, potentially leading to significant improvements in patient safety and care. The potential benefits of overcoming these challenges are immense and motivate people to continue their efforts in this field [7].

2. Challenges in PV systems in low- and middle-income countries

The integration and reliability of pharmacovigilance systems across LMICs remain limited despite recent efforts to harmonise PV rules and regulations in several regional economic communities.

2.1 Underreporting

The detection and prevention of ADRs is a critical aspect of pharmacovigilance, but significant challenges hinder it. Although spontaneous reporting is the most effective method for identifying new and rare ADRs, underreporting remains an important issue. Despite the widespread adoption of reporting systems and their benefits, ensuring that all ADRs are accurately reported is difficult. **Table 1** lists the reporting system/centre involved in the coordination of the PV activities in a few LMICs.

Sl. No	Reporting system	Country
1	Pharmacovigilance Programme of India (PvPI)	India
2	National Pharmacovigilance Centre (NPC)	Nigeria
3	South African Health Products Regulatory Authority (SAHPRA)	South Africa
4	National Agency of Drug and Food Control (BPOM)	Indonesia
5	Brazilian Health Regulatory Agency (ANVISA)	Brazil

Table 1.
Showing the reporting system name involved in the coordination of the PV activities, including the name of the country.

2.2 Pharmacovigilance training in LMIC

The shortage of professionals with specialised knowledge in PV is primarily due to the limited accessibility of specialised training programmes in this area. Although some institutions in selective locations provide PV training, most universities do not offer courses or educational programmes that cover a wide range of subjects related to PV. This lack of comprehensive education often results in graduates and employees having insufficient data collection and analytical skills. For harmonisation, it is required to adhere to the formatting standards of international or World Health Organisation (WHO) pharmacovigilance databases.

2.3 Funding constraints

PV activities in numerous LMICs rely mainly on external funds. Hence, they frequently face funding- and/or grant-related challenges. Salaries (remuneration) for people working in this sector are generally lower in these resource-constrained nations than in other sectors and contractual in a few countries like India. Also, ADR monitoring centres are not being supported financially to carry out any outreach activity and training programmes.

2.4 Public engagement

Failing to incorporate patients in a reporting strategy, particularly in underdeveloped nations where medications are often self-administered without medical supervision, may lead to underestimating critical data or significant delays in identifying early warning signs [8].

2.5 Reporting form

The inaccessibility and complexity of reporting forms pose challenges in some countries. Additionally, language barriers can present a significant obstacle when patients cannot report in their native language, particularly in countries with multiple local languages.

2.6 Regulation-related issues

Legislation and regulations related to drug safety in many developing countries, if they exist, are often perceived as insufficient and weak. This is evidenced by the pharmaceutical industry's lack of accountability for pharmacovigilance, as demonstrated by Moscou's research on the commitment of six multinational companies to pharmacovigilance internationally and in India. The study found that pharmacovigilance is not adequately integrated into the policies of the companies studied, particularly in their Indian subsidiaries.

2.7 Lack of confidentiality and fear of professional dignity attrition

Healthcare professionals may hesitate to report adverse drug reactions related to treatments for several reasons, including the fear of being perceived as incompetent or culpable, the absence of explicit legal provisions guaranteeing the confidentiality of submitted reports, and a lack of trust in the authorities involved.

2.8 Clinical trial limitations

Clinical trials are usually conducted for a limited period under strictly controlled conditions on a few carefully selected individuals who meet specific inclusion and exclusion criteria. The limited number of subjects in these trials can make detecting less common or rare events difficult, resulting in a lack of complete safety data for rational prescription.

2.9 Issues with attitudes towards ADR reporting

Lack of time from routine clinical activities. Physicians usually claim that managing ADRs is more critical than reporting them, and some people feel there is a lack of incentives for reporting them [9].

2.10 Complexity of healthcare system

Self-medication frequently constitutes a significant portion of overall medication usage. This phenomenon is partly attributed to the expenses of seeking professional medical assistance and the scarcity of trained healthcare providers, particularly in

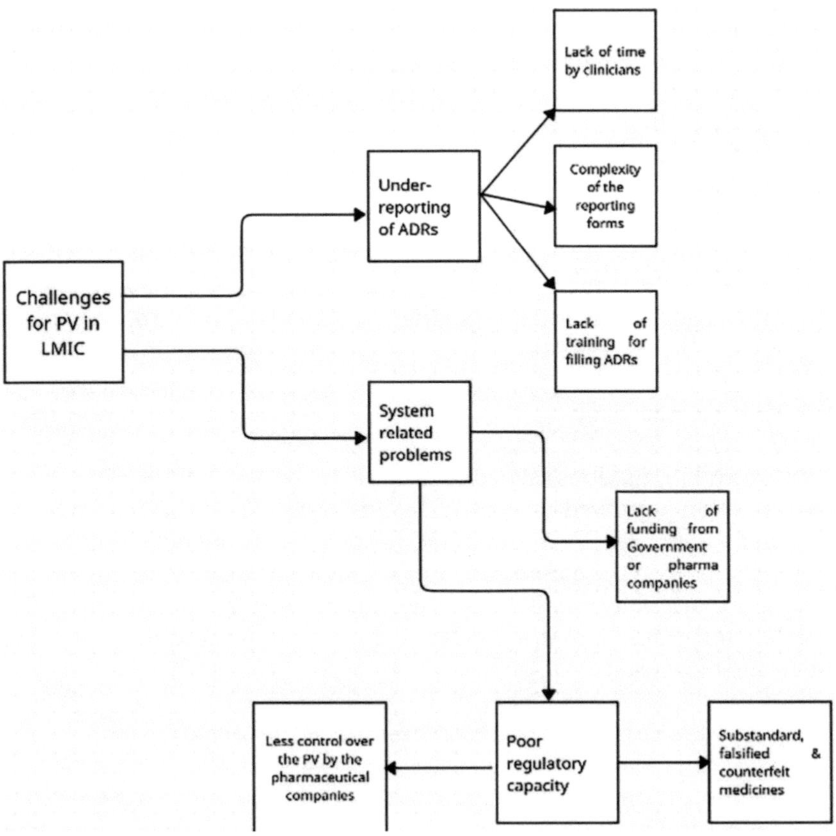

Figure 1.
Outlines the challenges for PV systems in LMIC.

rural and remote regions. As a result, individuals frequently resort to traditional healers or unlicensed vendors instead of relying on formal healthcare facilities.

2.11 Sentinel sites and active surveillance

In incorporating novel medications into public health programmes for unfamiliar populations, it is generally suggested to undertake sentinel site monitoring or active surveillance, such as cohort event monitoring. Although a select few countries have documented the employment of sentinel sites or active surveillance for pharmacovigilance, these studies are probably not being maximised to their full potential due to the necessity for specialised funding, systematic record-keeping, and expertise in methodology.

2.12 Insufficient national coordination of PV activities

Inadequate collaboration, coordination, and conflict of interest between major national PV stakeholders hinders PV development.

The challenges in PV systems in LMIC are summarised in **Figure 1**.

3. Consequences due to challenges in pharmacovigilance in LMIC

3.1 Delayed detection of drug safety issues

Poor PV systems delay detection and response to drug safety problems. Without timely and accurate reporting, it becomes difficult to identify and address the harmful effects of medications, which can lead to prolonged exposure of populations to unsafe drugs. This delay can result in increased morbidity and mortality among patients.

3.2 Increased risk of substandard and falsified medicines

Weak pharmacovigilance systems struggle to identify and address issues related to substandard, spurious, falsely labelled, and falsified medicines, posing significant public health risks [10].

3.3 Insufficient regulatory oversight

Inadequate regulatory oversight means that ADRs may not be systematically recorded or investigated, and necessary regulatory actions, such as drug recalls or label changes, may not be implemented promptly.

3.4 Increased mortality and morbidity

Ineffective PV in LMICs will result in increased mortality and morbidity associated with undetected ADRs and due to the continued use of unsafe medications.

3.5 Economic burden

The costs of managing ADRs, including additional medical treatments, hospitalisations, and productivity losses, can strain already limited healthcare budgets.

- Therapeutic ineffectiveness
- Development of antimicrobial resistance
- Inadequate safety data among the special population (e.g. pregnant women, children) because they are usually excluded in the clinical trial

4. Possible solutions

The following strategies in **Figure 2** are derived from international experiences and tailored to promote PV practices in LMICs. They have been selected based on their suitability in these specific contexts.

4.1 Educating HCPs

Strong technical knowledge can be an asset in successfully running a pharmacovigilance programme. HCPs' training techniques clarify the importance of reporting, and the procedures must be designed and implemented to stimulate reporting by all health team members [11]. Lectures, workshops, scientific meetings, conference sessions, printed educational materials, and publications in professional journals could all contribute to fostering a reporting culture among medical practitioners, ultimately leading to a notable rise in reporting rates [12]. Since 1993, the Uppsala Monitoring Centre (UMC) has started conducting an international pharmacovigilance training course in Uppsala, Sweden, and in recent years, also in Mysore, India. Recently, E-learning modules using a microlearning approach to allow for distance learning and to address technological challenges were developed, launched, and evaluated [13]. In addition, regular in-service training opportunities and easy-to-access updates on pharmacovigilance should be made available.

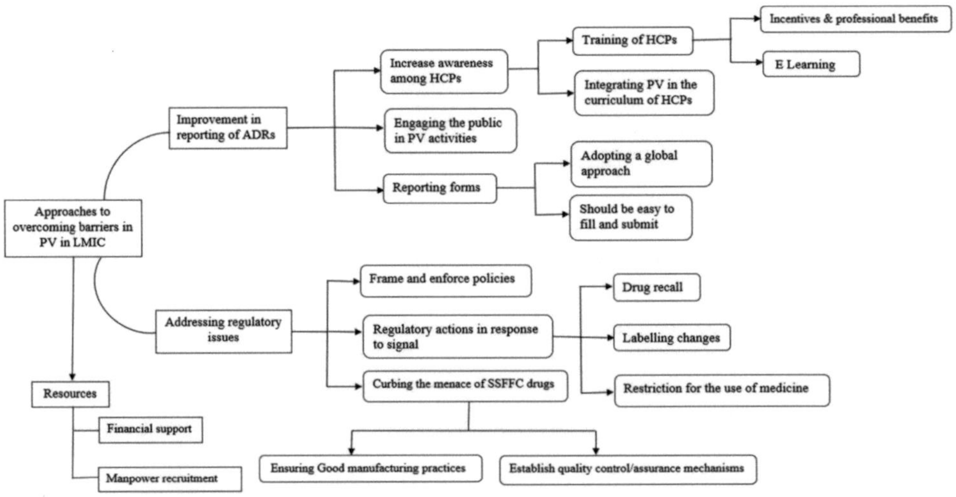

Figure 2.
Diagram illustrating strategies and approaches to overcome barriers in PV in LMIC (Part of the diagram is reproduced after permission from Elshafie S).

4.2 Feedback provided to healthcare workers, policymakers, and consumers in response to pharmacovigilance reports

Healthcare professionals receive detailed feedback on ADRs they report, which helps them recognise patterns, understand potential drug risks, and adjust treatment plans accordingly. Policymakers use aggregated data from these reports to formulate or modify drug safety regulations and public health policies, ensuring a more robust pharmacovigilance system. For consumers, feedback often includes information on the safety of medications, potential side effects, and guidance on reporting ADRs, empowering them to make informed decisions about their treatments and participate actively in the healthcare process.

4.3 Collaboration and partnerships

Collaboration between PV centres is essential for sharing information, establishing best practices in ADR monitoring, and enhancing the science of pharmacovigilance. The WHO emphasises the importance of multidisciplinary collaboration among health ministries, universities, NGOs, pharmaceutical industries, and other stakeholders to improve ADR monitoring activities. Additionally, partnerships with practitioner consortia specialising in specific types of ADRs, such as drug-induced liver injury, can provide detailed adverse event (AE) reports and interactions with clinicians. Furthermore, collaboration with community pharmacists can yield ADRs, as they are the first point of contact in the existing healthcare system.

4.4 Engaging the public

As drug safety surveillance systems advance, it is essential for them to continue prioritising the perspectives and needs of both patients and practitioners by providing valuable and actionable information about medicine safety and proper usage. However, many existing reporting methods tend to focus more on input from professionals rather than consumer self-reporting. Consumer reporting captures the ADRs caused by over-the-counter (OTC) medications, herbal medications, and medicines prescribed by unqualified professionals [14]. By incorporating consumer data, there is an opportunity to enhance the overall understanding of medication safety and detect potential ADRs earlier.

Disseminating information about reporting processes and utilising various media channels, such as newsletter articles, general media programmes, and sensitisation campaigns, can be effective strategies for increasing public awareness and engagement in reporting ADRs. This approach can foster a deeper understanding and recognition of the importance of reporting ADRs among the public.

4.5 Incorporation of informatics

Advances in the availability of data and analytic methods are transforming the field of pharmacovigilance. The transition from paper-based medical records to electronic healthcare records has increased interest in mining these data to detect drug safety signals. However, there are two significant limitations in the current pharmacovigilance data: minimal data on indications for use and minimal data on product identifiers. These limitations could be partially addressed by incorporating health informatics, such as the Hospital Information Management System (HIMS). In addition, standardised data on product identification would enable a better correlation of adverse event data with product quality data, bridging the gap between pharmacovigilance systems and product quality systems, which would be an essential step forward.

4.6 Leveraging modern technology

Online reporting and mobile phone applications, such as Med Safety App and WhatsApp, can be utilised to improve pharmacovigilance. For instance, the South African Mom-Connect platform demonstrates how technological advancements enable patient self-reporting by allowing pregnant women to input information about medication exposure and potential harm directly. Additionally, these advancements can support two-way communication between PV centres, patients, and practitioners, especially in regions with no other infrastructure. In this technically advanced, modernised world, India, under the Pharmacovigilance Programme of India (PvPI), has launched a mobile application, "ADR-PvPI", as a tool for ADR reporting [15].

4.7 Integrating PV in the curriculum of HCPs

There is a great need to introduce PV at the undergraduate and graduate levels in teaching institutions for all health professionals worldwide. Recently, India made it compulsory for all medical and pharmacy colleges to include PV training in the undergraduate curriculum [16].

4.8 Adopting a global approach

One component of a global approach is harmonisation, the process of establishing common technical standards across countries and regions with diverse legal and regulatory bases for drug regulation. From a global perspective, national PV systems should set up and maintain individual case safety report (ICSR) databases compatible with the international standard format for ICSR reports, the ICH-E2b. The global standard allows easy exchange of ICSRs between countries, regulatory authorities, and marketing authorisation holders (MAHs). Establishing E2b-compatible systems is expensive, but LMICs can utilise the Vigiflow data management system offered and maintained at a meagre cost by the UMC as it integrates E2b standards within it.

4.9 Project 3S (smart safety surveillance)

The WHO Safety and Vigilance (SAV) Team has initiated a project to optimise post-marketing surveillance of priority medicines and vaccines in LMICs. The project will use a smart safety surveillance ("3S") approach that initially focuses on selected priority products to be introduced in LMICs. As safety data will be generated on specific products in parallel with their first use, national pharmacovigilance systems and competence will be strengthened to enable safety monitoring of all products in the long term. Project 3S proposes strengthening, expanding, and streamlining pharmacovigilance systems in LMICs [17].

4.10 Artificial intelligence (AI)-based pharmacovigilance

AI-based pharmacovigilance detection, improving training and education, and informing the government of the benefits of AI-based pharmacovigilance help solve these challenges in settings with limited resources. However, the quantity and quality of data directly affect AI performance, and implementing AI in limited-resource settings presents challenges. Opportunities for improvement include collaborative research networks, pharmacogenomic research and practices, and advanced machine-learning algorithms [18].

4.11 Funding and financial sustainability of pharmacovigilance

The primary source of funding in resource-limited African countries is from the government, which provides significant donor funding that is ad hoc and non-sustainable. To ensure financial sustainability potential sources of funding have been identified, which include fees from commercialised services like user fees, registration, and licencing fees etc., PV tax on pharmaceutical sales, community financing, funds from pharma consortium and donor financing from WHO, United Nations International Children's Fund (UNICEF), The United States Agency for International Development (USAID), Bill and Melinda Gates Foundation (BMGF) can be explored. Enabling a legal framework that will engender autonomy will provide a sustainable mechanism for PV funding [19].

4.12 Incentives and professional benefits

Incentives in the form of continuing medical education (CME) credit points can be provided to medical professionals who undergo training in PV modules, and PV is made mandatory for the recognition of colleges for admitting the students in professional courses regulated by Pharmacy Council of India (PCI) and National Medical Council (NMC) in India.

4.13 Develop holistic PV strengthening plans

A holistic plan for pharmacovigilance will be developed in each country covering (1) policy, law, and regulation; (2) system, structure, and stakeholder coordination; (3) signal generation and data management; (4) risk assessment and evaluation; and (5) risk management, communication, and allocation of commensurate resources.

4.14 Targeted pharmacovigilance awareness campaigns in LMIC should leverage public health programmes (e.g. HIV, malaria, tuberculosis)

WHO has produced PV handbooks addressing the specific needs for PV in malaria, HIV/AIDS, and tuberculosis, focusing on cohort event monitoring and targeted spontaneous reporting. Many LMIC countries, for example, Ghana, Nigeria, Tanzania, Kenya, Uganda, and Zimbabwe, have piloted these methods and have demonstrated their feasibility.

4.15 Assessing impact

We need to assess the impact of an intervention on PV activities, which will help PV centres plan and allocate resources effectively. The WHO pharmacovigilance indicators assess the effectiveness of a country's PV system [20]. We also have pharmacovigilance indicators for public health programmes, which involve many people's exposure to medicinal products.

5. Conclusions

Low- and middle-income countries (LMICs) face unique challenges in establishing robust pharmacovigilance (PV) systems. Underreporting of adverse drug reactions (ADRs) remains a significant issue, even in jurisdictions where reporting is mandatory. The scarcity of professionals with expertise in PV, limited funding, lack of public engagement, inaccessibility to reporting forms, language barriers, and the complexity of the healthcare system contribute to the challenges. Regulation-related issues, such as insufficient legislation and weak accountability of the pharmaceutical industry, pose additional obstacles. Healthcare professionals may refrain from reporting ADRs due to fear of professional dignity attrition and the absence of explicit legal provisions ensuring confidentiality. Clinical trials have limitations in detecting rare events, and attitudes towards ADR reporting, such as lack of time and incentives, further complicate the situation. Despite these challenges, establishing robust PV systems in LMICs can generate valuable data to inform crucial healthcare policy and practice decisions, potentially leading to significant improvements in patient safety and care.

Acknowledgements

I want to thank IPC, Ghaziabad, the NCC for PVPI for providing technical support during my tenure as Deputy and Co-ordinator at AMCs in India.

Conflict of interest

The authors declare no conflict of interest.

Author details

Anant Khot* and Ganesh Dakhale
Department of Pharmacology, AIIMS, Nagpur, India

*Address all correspondence to: anantkhot04@gmail.com

IntechOpen

© 2024 The Author(s). Licensee IntechOpen. This chapter is distributed under the terms of the Creative Commons Attribution License (http://creativecommons.org/licenses/by/4.0), which permits unrestricted use, distribution, and reproduction in any medium, provided the original work is properly cited.

References

[1] Kumar A. Pharmacovigilance: Importance, concepts, and processes. American Journal of Health-System Pharmacy. 2017;**74**:e101-e107

[2] Swamy S, Mourya M, Kadhe G, Mane A, Sawant S. Safety reporting through a comprehensive and pragmatic pharmacovigilance process for India and emerging markets: An industry perspective. Expert Opinion on Drug Safety. 2015;**14**(9):1409-1420

[3] Olsson S, Pal SN, Dodoo A. Pharmacovigilance in resource-limited countries. Expert Review of Clinical Pharmacology. 2015;**8**(4):449-460

[4] Nguyen XH, Le TA, Nguyen AT, Thu T, Pham H, Tran TH. Supply chain risk, integration, risk resilience and firm performance in global supply chain: Evidence from Vietnam pharmaceutical industry. Uncertain Supply Chain Management. 2021;**9**:779-796

[5] Akel M, Ramia E, Hajj A, Hallit S, Lahoud N, Zaytoun A, et al. Medication safety spontaneous reporting system: The Lebanese order of pharmacists initiative. Bulletin of Faculty of Pharmacy Cairo University. 2019;**57**(1):66-72

[6] Elshafie S, Zaghloul I, Roberti AM. Pharmacovigilance in developing countries (part I): Importance and challenges. International Journal of Clinical Pharmacy. 2018;**40**(4):758-763

[7] Kiguba R, Olsson S, Waitt C. Pharmacovigilance in low- and middle-income countries: A review with particular focus on Africa. British Journal of Clinical Pharmacology. 2023;**89**:491-509

[8] Olsson S, Pal SN, Stergachis A, Couper M. Pharmacovigilance activities in 55 low-and middle-income countries a questionnaire-based analysis. Drug Safety. 2010;**33**(8):689-703

[9] Mulchandani R, Kakkar A. Reporting of adverse drug reactions in India: A review of the current scenario, obstacles, and possible solutions. The International Journal of Risk & Safety in Medicine. 2019;**30**(1):33-44

[10] Dal Pan GJ. Ongoing challenges in pharmacovigilance. Drug Safety. 2014;**37**(1):1-8

[11] Elshafie S, Roberti AM, Zaghloul I. Pharmacovigilance in developing countries (part II): A path forward. International Journal of Clinical Pharmacy. 2018;**40**(4):764-768

[12] Pagotto C, Varallo F, Mastroianni P. Impact of educational interventions on adverse drug events reporting. International Journal of Technology Assessment in Health Care. 2013;**29**(4):410-417

[13] Hegerius A, Caduff-Janosa P, Savage R, Ellenius J. E-learning in pharmacovigilance: An evaluation of microlearning-based modules developed by Uppsala Monitoring Centre. Drug Safety. 2020;**43**(11):1171-1180

[14] Palaian S. Pharmacovigilance practices and activities: Issues, challenges, and future direction. In: Ibrahim MIM, Wertheimer AI, Babar ZUD, editors. Social and Administrative Aspects of Pharmacy in Low- and Middle-Income Countries. London (UK): Academic Press; 2018. pp. 145-162

[15] Kalaiselvan V, Srivastava S, Singh A, Gupta S. Pharmacovigilance in India: Present scenario and future challenges. Drug Safety. 2019;**42**(3):339-346

[16] Menang O, Kuemmerle A, Maigetter K, Burri C. Strategies and interventions to strengthen pharmacovigilance systems in low-income and middle-income countries: A scoping review. BMJ Open. 2023;**13**(9):e071079. DOI: 10.1136/bmjopen-2022-071079

[17] Monika Z. Safety of medicines: Priming resource-limited countries for pharmacovigilance. WHO Drug Information. 2017;**31**(4):575-580

[18] Liang L, Hu J, Sun G, Hong N, Wu G, He Y, et al. Artificial intelligence-based pharmacovigilance in the setting of limited resources. Drug Safety. 2022;**45**:511-519. DOI: 10.1007/s40264-022-01170-7

[19] Isah AO, Opadeyi AO, Tumwijukye H, Cobelens F, Smith D, Ndomondo-Sigonda M, et al. Funding and financial sustainability of pharmacovigilance: Suggested models for funding pharmacovigilance in resource-limited African countries. Therapeutic Advances in Drug Safety. 2023;**14**:1-14

[20] Who Pharmacovigilance Indicators: A Practical Manual for the Assessment of Pharmacovigilance Systems. Geneva (Switzerland): WHO Press; 2015. pp. 4-15

Chapter 5

Perspective Chapter: Constant Need for Pharmacovigilance Improvement in Bosnia and Herzegovina

Martin Kondža

Abstract

Bosnia and Herzegovina is a county in South-East Europe with a complicated political structure. This political division led to a late formation of a national governing body on medicines and medical devices, as well as pharmacovigilance. Pharmacovigilance is currently under the jurisdiction of the Agency for Medicines and Medical Devices and its National Pharmacovigilance Office in Mostar. Looking at the organized pharmacovigilance systems in neighboring countries, recommendations for improving the pharmacovigilance system can be found. Such changes will result in significant improvements in public health and patient safety. When the pharmacovigilance system is efficient, it enables early identification and assessment of risks associated with the use of drugs. This leads to faster withdrawal or replacement of harmful drugs from the market, reducing the risk of serious side effects and potentially fatal outcomes. In addition, an improved system of pharmacovigilance promotes the confidence of patients and health professionals in the safety of medicines, which is essential for successful treatment. Education and training of healthcare workers on the importance of reporting side effects and the use of advanced technologies for data collection and analysis also play a key role in strengthening the system. The implementation of these measures will contribute to the creation of a safer health environment in Bosnia and Herzegovina.

Keywords: Bosnia and Herzegovina, pharmacovigilance, materiovigilance, medicines, ALMBIH

1. Introduction

Bosnia and Herzegovina (B&H) has a complex political structure that is the result of the General Framework Agreement for Peace in Bosnia and Herzegovina, a.k.a. *Dayton Peace Agreement*, signed in 1995 [1], which ended the war in B&H. The country's political structure is shaped as a decentralized state consisting of two entities: the Federation of Bosnia and Herzegovina (FB&H) and the Republic of Srpska (RS) as well as the Brčko District, which has a special status [2]. FB&H is further divided into 10 counties with their own jurisdiction in different areas. At the state level, B&H has a three-member Presidency consisting of three members, who should represent the three constituent nations of B&H [3]. This complex political structure not only reflects the ethnic and political diversity of B&H, but also creates challenges in terms of governance efficiency and political stability. Such a political structure further spills over into the spheres of social and professional life of all its citizens. This is also the situation with the healthcare system. In most countries of the world, the healthcare system is divided into several key institutions—the Ministry of Health, the Institute for Public Health and the Institute for Health Insurance. In B&H, the situation is significantly more complicated, when it is taken into account that every level of government—from the highest to the lowest has its own institutions of this type. In the country, there are more than 10 ministries that regulate the field of health, as many institutes for health insurance and several institutes for public health [2]. Therefore, the medicine policy is split between different ministries and institutes.

Until 2009, this area was mostly divided between two institutions in B&H. The regulation of drugs and medical devices in FB&H was under the jurisdiction of the Institute for Drug Control FB&H and the Institute for Public Health of the RS. May 1st, 2009 marked the establishment of the Agency for Medicines and Medical Devices of Bosnia and Herzegovina (Croatian *Agencija za lijekove i medicinska sredstva Bosne i Hercegovine*, ALMBIH) as the main body for the regulation, control and supervision of medicines at the state level. ALMBIH was founded on the basis of the Law on Medicines and Medical Devices of B&H [4] in order to ensure the availability of safe, high-quality and effective drugs and medical devices on the market of B&H. The jurisdiction of this state institution, which is responsible for its work to the Parliamentary Assembly of B&H, is limited to medicines, medical devices and vaccines in the territory of the entire B&H. In this way, ALMBIH took over the roles previously held by some other state bodies. It is geographically divided into three parts with offices in Sarajevo, Banja Luka and Mostar. ALMBIH carries out the procedure of registration of new drugs and medical devices before they can be placed on the market. This includes the assessment of product quality, safety and efficiency. The inspection control of medicines, vaccines and medical devices is a key component of the work of this institution in order to ensure the consistent quality of drugs and medical devices on the market. ALMBIH issues work permits to Marketing Authorization Holders (MAHs) to put medicines on the market and regulates this market in B&H and provides information to health workers and the public about the proper use of medicines and medical devices, especially in the form of letters to health workers about new knowledge about the safety and effectiveness of medicines. Moreover, ALMBIH is responsible for regulating all clinical trials that take place on the territory of B&H [4].

However, one of the most important roles of ALMBIH is the process of pharmacovigilance and materiovigilance; monitoring of side effects and safety of drugs, vaccines and medical devices after they are placed on the market. ALMBIH collects, analyzes and responds to reported side effects to ensure that the benefits of medicines outweigh the risks. The National Office for Pharmacovigilance and Materiovigilance is part of ALMBIH located in Mostar. This office systematically collects, analyzes, monitors and evaluates side effects collected through spontaneous reports submitted by health professionals (physicians, pharmacists, dentists, medical technicians and others), not only reports submitted by MAHs, but also reports received from MAHs around the world through the so-called CIOMS forms (Council for International Organizations of Medical Sciences) [5]. The work of the office is also focused on collecting periodical safety update reports (PSUR), cooperation with the World

Health Organization (WHO), Collaborative Center of the WHO at Uppsala—the Uppsala Monitoring Center (UMC), European Medicines Agency (EMA), its Pharmacovigilance Risk Assessment Committee (PRAC) and various other bodies. However, the work of this office has not been emphasized enough by the regulatory authorities for years, and it is clearly undercapacitated for all the necessary tasks that need to be performed. Therefore, such a situation is clearly reflected in the image of pharmacovigilance in B&H.

2. Pharmacovigilance and materiovigilance

There is probably no more significant event in the field of drug regulation than the thalidomide tragedy. The enormous failure of human civilization, the incalculable losses and destruction of human lives, but also the brave moves of a Canadian American doctor marked a turning point in the understanding of drug safety. From those events to the present day, a high standard for medicines has been set and civilizational progress has been made towards better, safer and more effective medicines. Pharmacovigilance (Greek *pharmakon*—drug and Latin *vigilare*—to keep watch) is the science and activities related to the detection, assessment, understanding and prevention of adverse effects or any other drug-related problems [6–9]. It plays a crucial role in ensuring that medicines are safe and effective for use, contributing significantly to public health [10, 11]. The primary goal of pharmacovigilance is to identify adverse drug reactions (ADRs) as early as possible, assess their significance and take action to minimize risks to patients [12]. This involves collecting and analyzing data from various sources, including clinical trials, spontaneous reports from healthcare professionals and patients, and scientific literature. The process of pharmacovigilance includes several key activities. Signal detection involves identifying new or previously unknown adverse effects from various data sources [12]. This is followed by signal evaluation, where the potential risk is assessed in terms of its frequency, severity and impact on patients. Risk management plans are then developed to minimize these risks, which may include updating product labels, issuing warnings or even withdrawing a drug from the market. Continuous monitoring ensures that any new information about a drug's safety profile is promptly acted upon.

Effective pharmacovigilance requires collaboration among regulatory authorities, pharmaceutical companies, healthcare professionals and patients. Regulatory bodies, such as the Food and Drug Administration (FDA) in the United States [13] and the EMA in Europe [14], play a pivotal role in overseeing pharmacovigilance activities. Pharmaceutical companies are responsible for monitoring the safety of their products and reporting any adverse events to the regulatory authorities. Healthcare professionals and patients are encouraged to report any suspected adverse drug reactions, which can provide valuable real-world data on a drug's safety. In recent years, advancements in technology have significantly enhanced pharmacovigilance practices. The use of electronic health records [15], big data analytics [16] and artificial intelligence [17] allows for more efficient detection and analysis of adverse drug reactions. These technologies enable the processing of vast amounts of data from diverse sources, improving the speed and accuracy of signal detection. Additionally, social media and online health communities have emerged as new sources of information on drug safety, providing insights into patient experiences that might not be captured through traditional reporting systems [18, 19].

A separate emerging trend is the pharmacovigilance of herbal remedies, which involves the systematic monitoring, evaluation and understanding of adverse effects and other safety-related issues associated with the use of herbal medicines. Herbal remedies, often perceived as natural and safe, can pose significant health risks due to factors, such as contamination, misidentification of plants, interactions with conventional medicines and variability in chemical composition. Therefore, robust pharmacovigilance practices are essential to ensure their safe use [20]. One of the primary challenges in the pharmacovigilance of herbal remedies is the lack of standardized regulations and quality control measures across different regions. Unlike conventional pharmaceuticals, herbal products may not always undergo rigorous clinical testing before being marketed. This can result in products of varying quality and efficacy, making it difficult to assess their safety profiles accurately. Establishing comprehensive regulatory frameworks and quality standards is crucial to address these issues and ensure the safety of herbal remedies [21].

Pharmacovigilance activities also play a crucial role in supporting patient safety during clinical trials. These activities ensure the protection of human subjects through oversight of informed consent processes, Institutional Review Board (IRB) approvals and data monitoring committees (DMCs). Establishing a drug's safety profile is another key function of pharmacovigilance, which involves assessing data from all phases of development, focusing on dose-limiting toxicities, maximum tolerated doses and adverse events of special interest [22]. Effective communication of safety information is crucial in pharmacovigilance. Pharmacovigilance ensures that key documents, such as the Investigator's Brochure, Company Core Data Sheet and regulatory submissions (e.g., US Prescribing Information (PI) and EU Summary of Product Characteristics), are maintained and updated. Post-marketing surveillance activities include monitoring for new adverse events and ensuring ongoing assessment of the benefit-risk balance [23].

In addition to monitoring clinical safety, pharmacovigilance oversees the safety of the manufacturing process. This includes conducting health hazard assessments for manufacturing deviations and addressing product complaints related to safety issues. Pharmacovigilance professionals develop and implement RMPs (Risk Management Plans) and REMS (Risk Evaluation and Mitigation Strategies) to manage identified risks, involving a comprehensive approach to understanding the product's risk profile and developing strategies to minimize these risks [24].

Materiovigilance (Greek *materia*—material and *vigilare* as mentioned above) is the systematic monitoring, evaluation and analysis of adverse incidents and other safety-related issues involving medical devices [25]. This specialized field of pharmacovigilance focuses on ensuring the safety, efficacy and performance of medical devices, ranging from simple tools like syringes to complex technologies like pacemakers and artificial hips [26]. The primary goal of materiovigilance is to identify and mitigate risks associated with medical devices to protect patient health and ensure that these products perform as intended [27]. The process of materiovigilance involves several critical activities, starting with the collection of data on adverse events and incidents related to medical devices. These data can come from various sources, including healthcare professionals, patients, manufacturers and regulatory bodies. Healthcare providers (HCPs) and patients play a crucial role in reporting any issues or malfunctions they encounter with medical devices. Such reporting is essential for identifying potential safety concerns and understanding the real-world performance of these devices [27].

Once adverse event reports are collected, the next step is to analyze and evaluate the data to identify any patterns or trends that might indicate a safety issue. This analysis involves assessing the severity, frequency and potential impact of the reported incidents. If a pattern is identified, it may signal a problem with a specific device or category of devices, prompting further investigation. Regulatory authorities and manufacturers work together to conduct these investigations, which may involve laboratory testing, clinical studies and consultations with experts. Risk management is a key component of materiovigilance. When a potential safety issue is identified, appropriate actions must be taken to mitigate the risks. These actions can include updating device labeling with new safety information, issuing warnings or recalls, modifying the design or manufacturing processes or even withdrawing the device from the market if necessary. The aim is to ensure that the benefits of using the medical device continue to outweigh any risks associated with its use [28].

Regulatory authorities play a central role in materiovigilance. Similar agencies as in pharmacovigilance (FDA, EMA) are responsible for overseeing the safety and effectiveness of medical devices. They establish regulations and guidelines for materiovigilance, ensuring that manufacturers comply with reporting requirements and maintain robust post-marketing surveillance systems. These regulatory bodies also collaborate internationally to share information and enhance global device safety. Technological advancements have significantly enhanced materiovigilance practices. The use of digital health technologies, electronic health records and big data analytics allows for more efficient and comprehensive monitoring of medical devices. These technologies enable the collection and analysis of large volumes of data from diverse sources, improving the ability to detect and respond to safety issues promptly. Additionally, artificial intelligence and machine learning can help identify patterns and predict potential device-related problems, further enhancing the effectiveness of materiovigilance [26].

Public awareness and education are also important aspects of materiovigilance. Informing healthcare professionals and patients about the importance of reporting adverse events and providing clear instructions on how to do so can improve the quality and quantity of data available for analysis. Transparent communication about the risks and benefits of medical devices helps build trust and ensures that users are well informed about the products they rely on for their health and well-being. Both pharmacovigilance and materiovigilance are critical aspects of healthcare that ensure the safety and efficacy of medical devices. Through systematic monitoring, analysis, risk management and regulatory oversight, materiovigilance helps protect patients from potential harm and ensures that medical devices deliver their intended benefits. As technology continues to evolve, materiovigilance practices will continue to improve, contributing to the ongoing enhancement of patient safety and public health.

2.1 Pharmacovigilance and materiovigilance system in B&H

The pharmacovigilance picture in B&H is not a good one. The National Office for Pharmacovigilance and Materiovigilance B&H in Mostar since the foundation of ALMBIH has had two full-time employees who do not have a higher education in the field of biomedical sciences, but a lower level of education. Due to the complex political situation, for a long time the Mostar center lacked pharmacy and medical professionals with the right skills and training. Add to that the absence of pharmacovigilance education among healthcare professionals, and one can see why B&H suffered from low adverse drug reaction (ADR) reporting numbers. Therefore, for years it was impossible to manage the key projects of this office and develop it to its full capacity. Certain changes occurred in 2017, when two external experts in the field of pharmacovigilance were hired to meet the needs of the office. The engagement of these experts, pharmacists by training, led to the implementation of a series of activities in the field of vigilance of drugs and medical devices. First of all, it started with the systematic recording of all received applications and the analysis of such applications by several categories. Applications were classified according to **Table 1** [29]:

After this type of classification, an individual assessment was made for each of the reported side effects and reviewed on the basis of the above classifications. All this resulted in a detailed individual report that was sent to each applicant and in which ALMBIH would, in accordance with legal regulations, provide its own safety assessment or intervene if necessary [4, 5]. Numerous campaigns were carried out in

Deployment	Classification
Based on type	Medicines Vaccines Medical devices
Based on status	Registered preparation Preparation from intervention import
Based on source	HCP • Physician • Physician-Specialist • Pharmacist • Nurse • Dentist • Pharmacy technician • Other HCPs MAH Public Health Institute
Based on seriousness	Serious • Death • Hospitalization or prolonged hospitalization • Permanent or severe disability or incapacity • Congenital anomaly • Life threatening • Medically serious condition Non-serious
Based on interactions	Drug or food interaction present • Concomitant medicines, herbal remedies or food Drug of food interaction excluded
Based on outcomes	Recovery without repercussions Recovery with repercussions Recovery ongoing Death
Cause-and-effect relationship	Certain Likely Possible Not likely

Table 1.
The deployment of adverse reactions to medicines, vaccines and medical devices and their classifications.

Healthcare Centers, hospitals, private clinics and other institutions. Initiatives have also been made for all tertiary-type healthcare institutions in B&H to appoint their own responsible person for pharmacovigilance affairs, in the same way as prescribed by law for MAH. The next initiative was related to professional institutions in the field of healthcare, primarily health chambers at all levels of government. Together with the leadership of these professional bodies, ALMBIH enabled changes to their own regulations, so that health workers received additional points for the renewal of health workers' licenses. Thus, positive relations were established with the Medical Chamber of FB&H, Chamber of Doctors of Medicine of RS, Pharmaceutical Chamber of FB&H, Pharmaceutical Chamber of RS, Dental Chamber of FB&H and Chamber of Doctors of Dentistry of RS. All these activities resulted in a huge increase in the number of applications. These activities have produced great results. In 2017, the center published its first annual ADR report, a collection of safety issues around medical products and medical devices gathered during the year. The number of ADR reports received in 2017 was the highest since the ALMBIH founding and represented an increase of 127% (to 283 total reports) compared to 2016. 2018 saw a 23% increase (to 349 total reports) compared to 2017, and a second annual report, with detailed data from 2018 followed. However, there were no public reports after this period, due to the external experts stopping with their work.

2.2 Reported ADRs

In its work, the National Center in Mostar relied on the decisions of competent authorities in the field of drug regulation, especially EMA, PRAC, Committee for Medicinal Products for Human Use (CHMP) and Coordination Group for Mutual Recognition and Decentralized Procedures—Human (CMDh), that is, the decision of the European Commission as the supreme authority for making binding decisions in the European Union (EU). Such decisions were revised and updated within B&H for the local area, to fully ensure the best possible protection of the population's health and the traceability of positive European decisions and regulations. In the regulation of the market of medicines and medical devices in B&H, the National Center very often followed the developments in neighboring countries and competent agencies for medicines, such as Croatia, Serbia and Montenegro.

In 2018, the National Center received 369 reports of suspected adverse effects of drugs and medical devices for processing and assessment in the field of drugs and medical devices. This number represents an increase of more than 30% compared to the figures from 2017, when the National Center received 283 reports of suspected adverse effects of drugs and medical devices. Therefore, 2018 represents the year with the largest number of applications received in B&H. Of the 369 applications received (**Figure 1**), 292 applications refer to medicines, while 77 applications refer to medical devices.

During 2018, the majority of applications received by the Main Office did not meet the criteria of seriousness (171), while 94 applications met the criteria of seriousness, namely in terms of hospital treatment or extension of hospital treatment (51), medically significant serious condition (31), threat to life (5), death (5) and permanent or severe disability or incapacity (2) (**Figure 2**).

When looking at the distribution of patients who experienced an ADR by gender, approximately equal numbers of male and female patients are observed (128 versus 124). For 12 patients, the gender is unknown (**Figure 3**). Such data are somewhat consistent with the relevant literature in this field, which talks about how women are the ones who experience more adverse drug reactions [31].

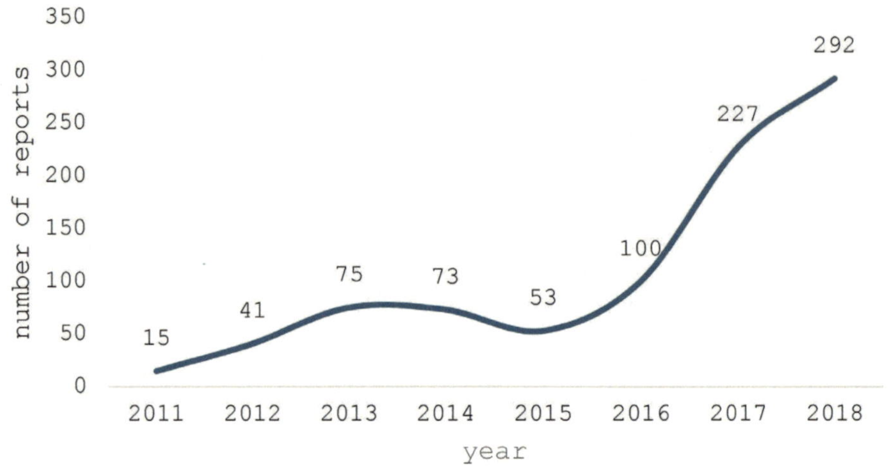

Figure 1.
Number of ADRs from 2011 to 2018 [30].

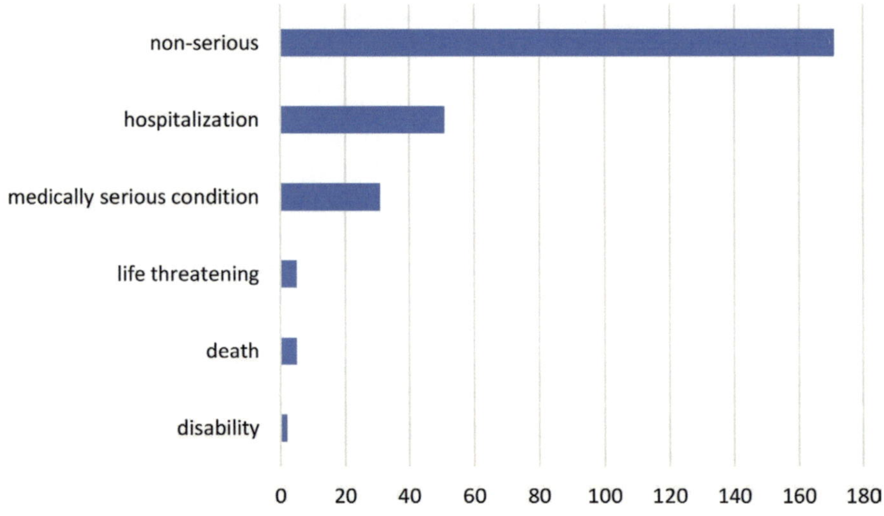

Figure 2.
ADR classification based on seriousness.

According to WHO-UMC recommendations and practice, patients can be divided into the following age groups:

- Premature ≤1 month
- Small child ≤4 years
- Child ≤11 years
- Adolescent ≤16 years
- Adults ≤69 years
- Elderly >69 years

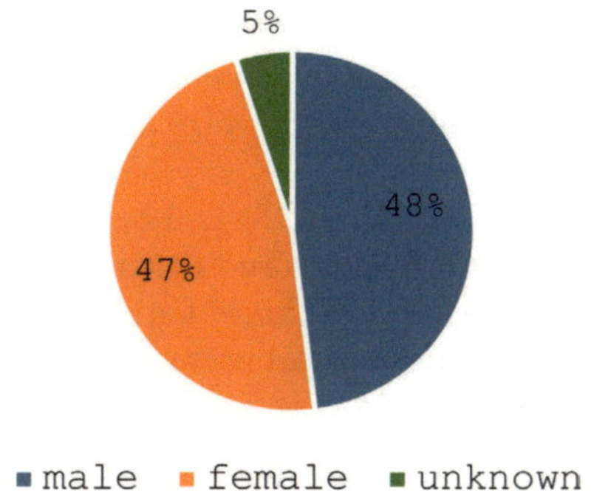

Figure 3.
Classification of patients based on sex.

ALMBIH is guided by the same classification according to age groups, and in 2018 it received the following applications, according to age groups: adults (176), elderly (32), small children (15), children (13) and adolescents (2) (**Figure 4**). The average age of the patient was 45 years.

In its daily work, the National Center uses the MedDRA (Medical Dictionary for Regulatory Activities) dictionary for regulatory affairs, a systematic dictionary of standardized medical terminology, created by the International Council for Harmonization (ICH). The MedDRA dictionary is intended for regulatory bodies, industry, research organizations, as well as healthcare professionals. Prior to the development of MedDRA dictionary, there was no internationally recognized, standardized medical terminology for regulatory affairs. The MedDRA dictionary consists of several levels of classification, with the highest level being system organ classification (SOC). The SOC level consists of 26 parts developed according to etiology, place of origin and purpose. The above SOC levels are further divided into preferred terms (PTs), which number over 20,000. Adverse drug effects should be displayed and grouped into PTs, since they best represent the adverse drug effect. Such PTs are then

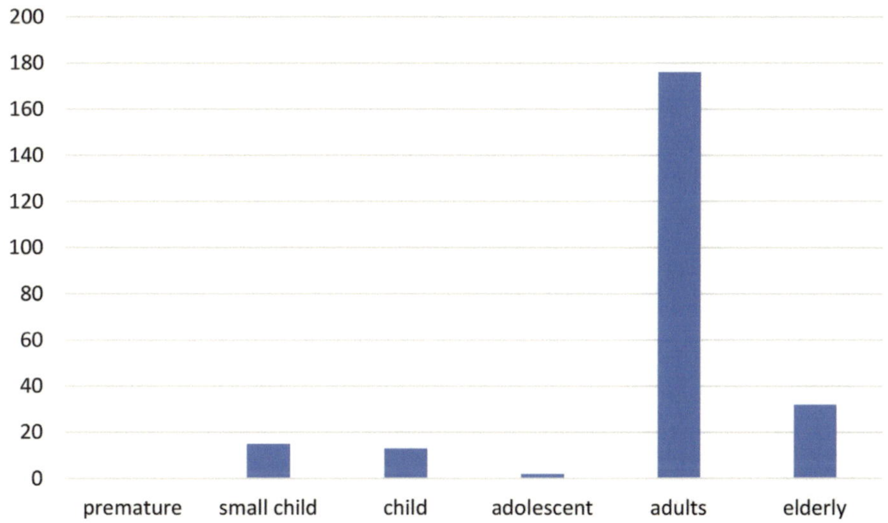

Figure 4.
Classification of patients based on age.

divided into lowest level terms (LLTs), of which there are over 70,000 [31]. The data for some of the most common ADRs at SOC level in 2018 are presented in **Table 2**.

PTs can give a slightly better picture of the very nature of the ADRs that have appeared (**Table 3**).

Most of the drugs that caused certain ADRs can be classified as drugs that are used for malignant diseases, immunomodulators and contrast agents (**Table 4**).

The pharmacovigilance system in B&H shows significant progress with an increase in the number of reports, which is the result of continuous work on raising awareness among healthcare workers and promoting the importance of reporting unwanted effects. However, there is still a need for further improvements to meet all WHO criteria.

2.3 HCPs as ADR reporters

In this process, healthcare professionals play a crucial role. Their primary responsibility includes recognizing and reporting suspected adverse drug reactions. Healthcare professionals, including doctors, pharmacists and nurses, are often the first to notice unusual drug reactions in patients. Their ability to accurately identify and document these side effects allows for rapid response and corrective action. In addition to recognizing side effects, healthcare professionals also have an educational role. They inform patients about the possible risks and side effects of prescribed drugs and the importance of reporting any adverse reactions. This is especially important for new drugs or those with a high risk of side effects. By informing and educating patients, healthcare professionals contribute to increasing awareness and cooperation in the pharmacovigilance process. Healthcare professionals also participate in research and studies that contribute to the understanding of the safety profile of drugs. Their clinical experience and daily work with patients provide invaluable insights that help them identify patterns of side effects and potential risks. Through these activities, healthcare professionals not only advance the science of drug safety, but also directly contribute to protecting the health of patients.

In B&H, doctors report the highest number of side effects to both drugs and medical devices. In the next place are pharmacists, then nurses (**Figure 5**).

The physicians who reported ADRs were mostly clinical pharmacologists, clinical radiologists, physicians with specialization in family medicine and pediatrics. Among

SOC class	Number of reports
Skin and subcutaneous tissue disorders	44
Gastrointestinal disorders	34
Immunological disorders	27
General disorders and administration site conditions	25
Infections and infestations	19
Nervous system disorders	19
Eye disorders	16
Respiratory, thoracic and mediastinal disorders	14
Blood and lymphatic system disorders	14

Table 2.
SOC classification of reported ADRs in 2018.

PT class	Number of reports
Urticaria	29
Anaphylaxis	26
Nausea	11
Abdominal pain	9
Colitis caused by *Clostridium difficile*	7
Uveitis	6
Erythema	5
Headache	4
Bleeding	4
Diarrhea	4

Table 3.
Reported ADRs at PT levels.

Medicines under suspicion	Number of reports
Adalimumab	23
Iopromide	20
Rituximab	9
Pazopanib	9
Nilotinib	8
Phenoxymethylpenicillin	7
Etoposide	6
Iomeprol	6
Pregabalin	6
Sunitinib	6

Table 4.
Most common medicines that caused ADRs.

healthcare professionals, physicians are the ones who report the most side effects for several key reasons. First, they have access to detailed information about patients, their medical conditions and the treatments they are receiving, enabling them to identify and report side effects following the administration of drugs or therapies. As the most responsible for treating patients, physicians are specially trained to recognize and respond to side effects, as their education includes a deep understanding of pharmacology and possible drug interactions [32]. In addition, doctors often have the most direct contact with patients and follow them over long periods of time, which allows them to see changes in health that could be related to side effects. They are also aware of their legal and ethical responsibility for patient safety, so reporting side effects is part of their professional obligation [33]. In many healthcare systems, physicians are the primary users of adverse event reporting systems and have access to the appropriate tools and resources to do so. Patients still often contact their doctors first when they feel an unusual reaction to a drug, so doctors are the first to learn about potential side effects and can report them to the authorities [34].

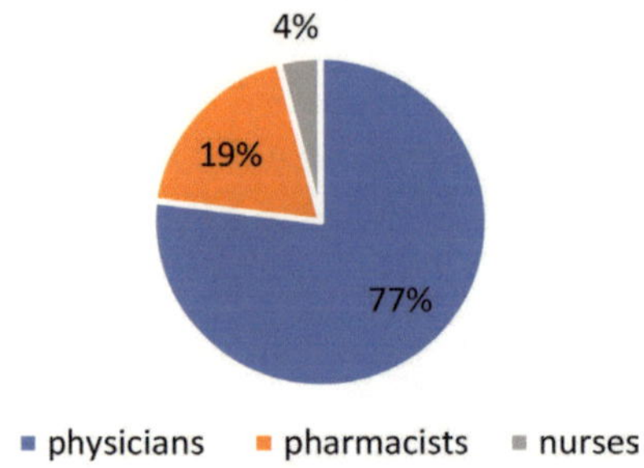

Figure 5.
HCPs as spontaneous reporters.

Pharmacists submitted 19% of the total reports in 2018. Pharmacists are often the first line of defense when it comes to reporting side effects. Because they are easily accessible and often in direct contact with patients, pharmacists are in a unique position to quickly identify and report side effects that patients experience. Their availability and proximity to patients enables a timely reaction to side effects, which is crucial for the prevention of more serious health problems [35].

In addition, pharmacists have specific knowledge about medicines, their mechanisms of action and possible side effects. This expertise allows pharmacists to recognize side effects that other healthcare professionals may not immediately spot. Their ability to distinguish between different types of side effects and to assess their significance contributes to the accuracy and relevance of reported data. Patient education is another important aspect of the pharmacist's role. Pharmacists are often the first source of information for patients about potential side effects of the medications they are taking. Through patient education, pharmacists ensure that patients are aware of the importance of reporting any unexpected or adverse drug reactions. Informed patients are better prepared to recognize and report side effects, which contributes to better drug safety monitoring [36].

Pharmacists can help prevent serious adverse drug reactions, which contributes to overall patient safety. Their role in reporting side effects is essential to protect patients and ensure that problems are identified and addressed in a timely manner. By reporting side effects, pharmacists in B&H help collect data that are necessary to assess the safety of drugs and make decisions about their further use.

2.4 Future recommendations

Although B&H and neighboring countries used to be part of the same state and the same drug control system, today in the era of independence there are significant differences in the number of side effects recorded, as well as the way of managing pharmacovigilance and the approach to this problem. One of the main reasons is the difference in the development and capacities of national drug agencies. In B&H, ALMBIH faces a lack of resources and employees dedicated to pharmacovigilance. The lack of financial resources and specialized training for healthcare workers further complicates the effective collection and management of side effects. In contrast, Croatia, which has a longstanding tradition in pharmacovigilance and significantly better resources, successfully conducts continuous education and develops advanced reporting systems [37].

An important reason is the different level of awareness and education about the importance of reporting side effects among healthcare professionals and patients.

Indicator	B&H	Croatia	Serbia	Montenegro
Public ADR reports	–	+	+	+
Points for HCP	+	+	+	+
Online reporting system	–	+	+	+
Mobile app for reporting	–	+	–	–
Patient can report ADR	–	+	+	+
Membership in WHO-UMC	+	+	+	+
WHO standards met	–	+	+	+

Table 5.
Differences in countries in terms of existing (+) or non-existing (−) pharmacovigilance indicators.

In B&H, a low percentage of applicants was recorded due to lack of education and somewhat complex application procedures. In Croatia, continuous education and promotion of pharmacovigilance, including innovative ways of reporting such as mobile applications, have significantly increased the number of reports, in such a way that Croatia is at the very top of Europe in terms of the number of reported side effects [38]. **Table 5** shows some of the differences in the pharmacovigilance systems of B&H and neighboring countries with the latest data [39–43].

An additional reason is the regulatory framework and implementation of the law. Although B&H has similar regulations as neighboring countries, their implementation and application are not at the same level. Croatia, for example, regularly publishes annual reports on pharmacovigilance and has a well-developed system for reporting side effects, including reporting by patients, which is not the case in B&H. Further differences are in the characteristics of the applicants. In Croatia, the percentage of applicants from among patients was significant, with a constant increase over the years, while patients in B&H cannot be applicants according to the current laws. Croatia also had a significantly higher percentage of applicants from the ranks of pharmacists compared to B&H and Montenegro [37].

Recommendations for the improvement of this area in B&H can be clearly read from the examples made by the neighboring countries. The first thing is the need to publish publicly available annual reports on the side effects of drugs, vaccines and medical devices. Publication of annual reports increases transparency and public trust in the healthcare system. When information about the side effects of drugs and medical devices is available to the public, patients and healthcare professionals can be more confident about the safety of the drugs they use. Transparency in the reporting and management of side effects also encourages the accountability of drug manufacturers and regulatory authorities [44]. Publicly available reports enable better information and education of healthcare workers. Physicians, pharmacists and other HCPs can use this information to identify and prevent potential risks associated with drug use. This increases patient safety and treatment efficiency, as informed healthcare professionals can make better decisions based on current data. In addition, the publication of the report encourages the more active participation of patients in their own healthcare. When patients are informed about possible drug side effects, they can more easily recognize and report them, thus contributing to the improvement of the entire pharmacovigilance system. Empowered patients can better manage their treatment and make informed decisions in collaboration with their doctors.

Since the reports for 2017 and 2018 were made and published, ALMBIH has experienced a halt in the process of publishing public reports on this topic. This approach is contrary to the valid legal provisions on which the ALMBIH also rests. Although spontaneous reports are regularly forwarded to the WHO-UMC database, it is necessary to work more on the transparency of this system, public visibility and raising awareness of the importance of pharmacovigilance and materiovigilance for this country. After this period, only one piece of information about adverse reactions to drugs and vaccines was published on the official website of ALMBIH, without indicating the classification of such drugs and vaccines. This move was probably the result of the emergence of the vaccine against the coronavirus disease 2019 (COVID-19) and the public's interest in the side effects of such vaccines. As stated on the official website of ALMBIH [45]: "*Since April 2019, the Agency for Medicines and Medical Devices of Bosnia and Herzegovina has been a full member of the Uppsala Monitoring Center network of national pharmacovigilance centers and is the only institution from Bosnia and Herzegovina that has access to the WHO-UMC database in which reports of adverse drug reactions from all over the world are forwarded. By December 31, 2022, a total of 1,680 reports were submitted to the WHO-UMC database for global monitoring of adverse drug reactions from Bosnia and Herzegovina. Compared to 2021, in 2022 the number of received reports of unwanted drug effects increased, while reports of COVID-19 vaccines were received in a reduced volume until July 2022. The sector for pharmacovigilance and materiovigilance of ALMBIH in the period from January 1st until December 31st 2022 received a total of 311 reports, of which: 284 reports of adverse drug reactions and 27 reports of reactions to vaccines*" (**Table 6**).

On the official ALMBIH webpage, it is also stated that [45]: "*In the WHO-UMC database for global monitoring of adverse drug reactions from Bosnia and Herzegovina in 2022, a total of 543 reports for drugs and vaccines were reported, which included applications that were not previously reported in the WHO-UMC database, and were submitted from the authorization holder, after it has been established that there are no globally double-reported cases by the authorization holder*". Although the publication of any official data related to pharmacovigilance and materiovigilance is commendable, it must be emphasized that the publication of such reports is not of great importance for the improvement of this system in Bosnia and Herzegovina. Therefore, the professional leadership of ALMBIH in this area is proposed to compile and publish detailed reports that will include the exact number of drugs, vaccines and medical devices responsible for side effects, the appropriate classification of these preparations, the exact source of reports, the results of reports, as well as the sociological profile of patients who were exposed to side effects.

The publication of detailed reports on the side effects of drugs, vaccines and medical devices has multiple advantages that can significantly improve not only the health and safety of patients, but also the entire healthcare system in B&H. The first and most

Indicator	Number of reports
Total number of reports	311
Reports on medicines	284
Report on vaccines	27
Regular immunization	6
COVID vaccines reports	21

Table 6.
Official ALMBIH pharmacovigilance and materiovigilance reports after 2018 [45].

important advantage is transparency. When the reports are detailed, including the classification of drugs, patients and primary sources of side effects, patients and healthcare professionals get a complete and clear picture of the safety of individual preparations. This allows patients to make informed decisions about their health and gives doctors the tools to prescribe therapies more precisely. Furthermore, detailed reports help identify patterns of side effects. When side effects are systematically monitored and documented, it is possible to observe certain trends or specific problems related to certain drugs or vaccines. This is particularly important for public health, as it enables rapid reaction and adjustment of treatment protocols, as well as withdrawal of dangerous preparations from the market if necessary. For example, if a particular drug is found to cause serious side effects in a particular population group, measures can be taken to protect that group.

Detailed reports also increase public confidence in the healthcare system and regulators such as ALMBIH. Transparency and openness in communication about the safety of medicines and medical devices increase the confidence of citizens that their health needs are taken seriously and that it is done in their best interest. Trust in the health system is critical to the successful implementation of health programs, including vaccination campaigns and other public health initiatives.

In order to maximize the benefits of detailed reports, ALMBIH should adopt several key recommendations. First, continuous and systematic collection of data on side effects should be ensured. This includes establishing reliable channels for reporting side effects by healthcare professionals and patients. Also, it is important to provide adequate training and support for all participants in this process in order to ensure accuracy and consistency of data. Reports should be published regularly and be easily accessible to the public. In the digital age, it is important that such information is available online, with the ability to search and analyze the data. This not only increases transparency, but also enables researchers, healthcare professionals and decision makers to use these data to improve healthcare practices further. ALMBIH should establish clear standards for classification and presentation of data. This includes detailed classification of drugs, vaccines and medical devices, as well as patients and types of side effects. The standardization of these data enables easier comparison and analysis, both within the country and internationally.

Čatić and Begović [46] also recognize the problem of lack of reporting and poor pharmacovigilance systems in B&H as a crucial one [46]. Underreporting of adverse drug reactions by healthcare workers is a major problem in many countries, including Bosnia and Herzegovina. In order to determine whether the pharmacovigilance system can be improved and to identify the reasons for underreporting, a study was conducted on the role of healthcare workers in reporting adverse drug reactions. The research showed that 62.9% of healthcare workers would report an adverse event to ALMBIH, but only 15.4% of respondents actually reported an adverse event. The majority of respondents have a positive perception about reporting side effects, but insufficient knowledge and experience in pharmacovigilance. The lack of experience in filling out the forms for reporting side effects and the inaccessibility of these forms were cited as the main obstacles to reporting. Reporting side effects is also perceived as time-consuming and complex. The authors emphasize the need for education and training of healthcare workers on pharmacovigilance, especially on the objectives of pharmacovigilance, filling in adverse reaction reporting forms and reporting criteria, as well as improving the adverse reaction reporting system in B&H [46].

Amrain and Bečić [47] found similar data in their research on pharmacists and family medicine doctors. Although both professional segments recognized the importance of pharmacovigilance, most of them did not report any side effects in 2014. The main barriers to reporting adverse events for pharmacists were the complexity of the reporting process, uncertainty and fear of misreporting, while physicians cited a lack of information about who to report an adverse event as the main barrier. Although healthcare professionals had a positive attitude towards reporting side effects, the reporting rate in B&H remains low. Various barriers to registration have been identified, and there is a need to improve traditional education in this area [47].

Regular publication of annual reports enables monitoring and analysis of trends in adverse drug reactions over time. These data are crucial for identifying new and rare side effects that may not have been detected during pre-marketing clinical trials. Also, they enable the evaluation of the effectiveness of existing safety measures and the adaptation of regulatory policies to improve the safety of medicines. Publicly available reports facilitate international cooperation and exchange of information with other countries and global pharmacovigilance authorities. This collaboration is essential for the rapid identification and resolution of safety issues on a global scale and contributes to the better protection of patient health worldwide.

Another key step may be to amend the current legislation in B&H to allow patients to report ADRs. Such legal regulations are currently in force in most European countries. Involving patients in reporting side effects increases the number and variety of reports, thereby improving the overall drug safety surveillance. Patients may often notice side effects that may not be obvious or may not be noted by healthcare professionals. Their reports add valuable data that help to understand better the effects of drugs under real conditions of use. Patients who are actively involved in reporting side effects become better informed about the potential risks and safety measures associated with the drugs they are using. This increases their awareness and enables them to be active participants in their own treatment, which can lead to better treatment outcomes and a reduced risk of serious side effects [48].

A system that allows patients to report side effects may reveal new or rare side effects that were not observed during clinical trials. Clinical trials often involve limited numbers of participants and specific conditions, while actual drug use may reveal different or additional side effects. Patient reports can help in the early detection of these problems and enable a faster response from regulatory authorities. Patients are given a voice in the drug safety monitoring process, which can increase trust in the healthcare system. When patients see that their reports have an impact and that steps are being taken to improve drug safety, they feel valued and are more motivated to continue participating in pharmacovigilance [49].

The third possibility refers to the online side effect reporting system and the mobile application for side effects. In order to implement this step, it is necessary to implement the previous step, that is, to enable wider communities of people to participate in the process of reporting side effects. A mobile application can make the process of reporting side effects much easier for patients and healthcare professionals. Smartphone use is widespread, and the app provides an easy and fast way to report side effects, anytime, anywhere. This can result in more reports and better drug safety monitoring. A mobile application can improve the quality of collected data. The application may include predefined forms and guides that guide users through the application process, ensuring that all required information is entered correctly. Also, the application can enable the sending of photographs and other relevant documents, thereby further enriching the database [50].

The application can provide users with instant feedback and educational content. After reporting a side effect, users can receive information on next steps or advice on how to proceed. Also, the application can contain educational modules on the recognition of side effects and the importance of reporting them, thereby increasing user awareness and knowledge. Also, this system enables better analytics and monitoring of trends in real time. The data collected through the application can be automatically analyzed and displayed in the form of statistics and graphs, which allows regulatory authorities to make decisions more quickly and efficiently. These analytics can help identify patterns and potential security issues faster than traditional methods [51].

3. Conclusion

The pharmacovigilance system in B&H faces numerous challenges due to the country's complex political structure and lack of resources. The National Office for Pharmacovigilance and Materiovigilance, located in Mostar, although it has achieved certain successes, continues to suffer from a lack of professional staff and financial resources. Despite these challenges, the increase in the number of adverse event reports in recent years shows that there is an awareness of the importance of pharmacovigilance among healthcare professionals. In order to improve the pharmacovigilance system in B&H, it is necessary to introduce several key measures. First, publishing publicly available annual reports on side effects of drugs, vaccines and medical devices would increase transparency and public trust in the healthcare system. Second, legislative changes that would allow patients to report side effects could significantly increase the number and variety of reports, thereby improving the overall drug safety monitoring. Third, the introduction of a system for online reporting of side effects and a mobile application would facilitate the reporting process for patients and healthcare workers, and enable faster and more efficient data analysis. The implementation of these measures requires political will, financial resources and continuous education of health workers and patients. Also, cooperation with international organizations such as the WHO and EMA can provide additional support and resources needed to improve the pharmacovigilance system in BiH. In this way, B&H can achieve a higher standard of drug safety, which will result in better protection of patients' health and greater trust in the healthcare system.

Acknowledgements

Prof. Dr. Kondža is the sole author of the manuscript. He has received no funding for the preparation of the manuscript.

Conflict of interest

The author declares no conflict of interest.

Thanks

The author would like to thank the Head of ALMBIH, Mrs. Nataša Grubiša, Prim, MPharm, and the Assistant Director for the Medicines Sector, Associate Professor Biljana Tubić, PhD, Spec, MPharm for their incredible dedication and brave work to improve the pharmaceutical system in Bosnia and Herzegovina as well as the health and well-being of all of its citizens.

Author details

Martin Kondža
Faculty of Pharmacy, University of Mostar, Mostar, Bosnia and Herzegovina

*Address all correspondence to: martin.kondza@farf.sum.ba

IntechOpen

© 2024 The Author(s). Licensee IntechOpen. This chapter is distributed under the terms of the Creative Commons Attribution License (http://creativecommons.org/licenses/by/4.0), which permits unrestricted use, distribution, and reproduction in any medium, provided the original work is properly cited.

References

[1] Organization for Security and Co-operation in Europe—OSCE. Dayton peace agreement. [Internet]. 1995. Available from: https://www.osce.org/bih/126173 [Accessed: May 15, 2024]

[2] Office of the High Representative—OHR.Constitution of Bosnia and Herzegovina. [Internet]. 1995. Available from: https://www.ohr.int/dayton-peace-agreement/annex-4/ [Accessed: May 16, 2024]

[3] Predsjedništvo Bosne i Hercegovine. Predsjedništvo. [Internet]. 2024. Available from: http://www.predsjednistvobih.ba/nadl/default.aspx?id=10005&langTag=bs-BA [Accessed: May 16, 2024]

[4] Parliament of Bosnia and Herzegovina. Law on medicines and medical devices. Official Gazette of Bosnia and Herzegovina. 2009;**58/08**

[5] Ministry of Civil Affairs of Bosnia and Herzegovina. Rulebook on the method of reporting, collecting and monitoring of adverse reactions to medicines in Bosnia and Herzegovina. Official Gazette of Bosnia and Herzegovina. 2012;**58/12**

[6] Kugener VF, Freedland ES, Maynard KI, Aimer O, Webster PS, Salas M, et al. Enhancing pharmacovigilance from the US experience: Current practices and future opportunities. Drug Safety. 2021;**44**(8):843-852. DOI: 10.1007/s40264-021-01078-8

[7] Lasys T, Santa-Ana-Tellez Y, Siiskonen SJ, Groenwold RHH, Gardarsdottir H. Unintended impact of pharmacovigilance regulatory interventions: A systematic review. British Journal of Clinical Pharmacology. 2023;**89**(12):3491-3502. DOI: 10.1111/bcp.15874

[8] Zatovkaňuková P, Slíva J. Diverse pharmacovigilance jurisdiction-the right way for global drug safety? European Journal of Clinical Pharmacology. 2024;**80**(3):305-315. DOI: 10.1007/s00228-023-03608-y

[9] Bouquet É, Star K, Jonville-Béra AP, Durrieu G. Pharmacovigilance in pediatrics. Therapie. 2018;**73**(2):171-180. DOI: 10.1016/j.therap.2017.11.012

[10] Bagheri H, Laroche ML, Montastruc JL. Pharmacovigilance: The new challenges. Therapie. 2016;**71**(2):121-122. DOI: 10.1016/j.therap.2016.02.019

[11] Dylan Fernandes S, Anoop NV, Castelino LJ, Narayana CR. A national approach to pharmacovigilance: The case of India as a growing hub of global clinical trials. Research in Social & Administrative Pharmacy. 2019;**15**(1):109-113. DOI: 10.1016/j.sapharm.2018.03.061

[12] Beninger P. Signal management in pharmacovigilance: A review of activities and case studies. Clinical Therapeutics. 2020;**42**(6):1110-1129. DOI: 10.1016/j.clinthera.2020.03.018

[13] Sakaeda T, Tamon A, Kadoyama K, Okuno Y. Data mining of the public version of the FDA adverse event reporting system. International Journal of Medical Sciences. 2013;**10**(7):796-803. DOI: 10.7150/ijms.6048

[14] Bakker E, Plueschke K, Jonker CJ, Kurz X, Starokozhko V, Mol PGM. Contribution of real-world evidence in European medicines agency's regulatory decision making. Clinical Pharmacology and Therapeutics. 2023;**113**(1):135-151. DOI: 10.1002/cpt.2766

[15] Kim SH. Active pharmacovigilance of drug-induced liver injury using electronic health records. Allergy Asthma & Immunology Research. 2020;**12**(3):378-380. DOI: 10.4168/aair.2020.12.3.378

[16] Trifirò G, Sultana J, Bate A. From big data to smart data for pharmacovigilance: The role of healthcare databases and other emerging sources. Drug Safety. 2018;**41**(2):143-149. DOI: 10.1007/s40264-017-0592-4

[17] Salas M, Petracek J, Yalamanchili P, Aimer O, Kasthuril D, Dhingra S, et al. The use of artificial intelligence in pharmacovigilance: A systematic review of the literature. Pharmaceutical Medicine. 2022;**36**(5):295-306. DOI: 10.1007/s40290-022-00441-z

[18] Tricco AC, Zarin W, Lillie E, Jeblee S, Warren R, Khan PA, et al. Utility of social media and crowd-intelligence data for pharmacovigilance: A scoping review. BMC Medical Informatics and Decision Making. 2018;**18**(1):38. DOI: 10.1186/s12911-018-0621-y

[19] Ravoire S, Lang M, Perrin E, participants of Giens XXXII Round Table No. 6. Advantages and limitations of online communities of patients for research on health products. Therapie. 2017;**72**(1):135-143. DOI: 10.1016/j.therap.2016.11.058

[20] Kondža M, Tubić B. Pharmacovigilance for herbal and traditional medicines in Bosnia and Herzegovina. In: Barnes J, editor. Pharmacovigilance for Herbal and Traditional Medicines: Advances, Challenges and International Perspectives. 1st ed. Auckland: Adis Cham; 2022. pp. 297-305. DOI: 10.1007/978-3-031-07275-8

[21] Brantley SJ, Argikar AA, Lin YS, Nagar S, Paine MF. Herb-drug interactions: Challenges and opportunities for improved predictions. Drug Metabolism and Disposition. 2014;**42**(3):301-317. DOI: 10.1124/dmd.113.055236

[22] White MG. Why human subjects research protection is important. The Ochsner Journal. 2020;**20**(1):16-33. DOI: 10.31486/toj.20.5012

[23] Gamble C, Wolf A, Sinha I, Spowart C, Williamson P. The role of systematic reviews in pharmacovigilance planning and clinical trials authorisation application: Example from the SLEEPS trial. PLoS One. 2013;**8**(3):e51787. DOI: 10.1371/journal.pone.0051787

[24] Esslinger S, Quinn L, Sampat S, Otero-Lobato M, Noël W, Geldhof A, et al. Risk management plans: Reassessment of safety concerns based on good pharmacovigilance practices module V (revision 2)-a company experience. Journal of Pharmaceutical Health Care and Sciences. 2022;**8**(1):14. DOI: 10.1186/s40780-022-00244-z

[25] Singh A, Jain M, Kapadia R, Advani U, Mahawar DK, Kakkar S, et al. Overview of materiovigilance programme of India. The RMJ. 2022;**16**(4):8-15

[26] Saifuddin PK, Tandon M, Kalaiselvan V, Suroy B, Pattanshetti V, Prakash A, et al. Materiovigilance programme of India: Current status and way forward. Indian Journal of Pharmacology. 2022;**54**(3):221-225. DOI: 10.4103/ijp.ijp_837_21

[27] Sapkota B, Palaian S, Shrestha S, Ibrahim MIM. Materiovigilance in perspective: Understanding its concept and practice in the global healthcare system. Therapeutic Innovation & Regulatory Science. 2023;**57**(4):886-898. DOI: 10.1007/s43441-023-00514-4

[28] Attri LK, Subhash Chandra BJ, Ramesh M, Chalasani SH, Syed J, Pal N. Materiovigilance in intensive care units: An active surveillance. Hospital Pharmacy. 2023;**58**(4):382-388. DOI: 10.1177/00185787221144931

[29] ALMBIH. First report on adverse reactions of medicines and medical devices. [Internet]. 2018. Available from: https://almbih.gov.ba/wp-content/uploads/2023/10/Izvjestaj_nezeljena_dejstva_2017.pdf [Accessed: May 20, 2024]

[30] ALMBIH. Second report on adverse reactions of medicines and medical devices. [Internet]. 2018. Available from: https://almbih.gov.ba/wp-content/uploads/2023/10/Izvjestaj_nezeljena_dejstva_2018.pdf [Accessed: May 20, 2024]

[31] Zhang X, Feng Y, Li F, Ding J, Tahseen D, Hinojosa E, et al. Evaluating MedDRA-to-ICD terminology mappings. BMC Medical Informatics and Decision Making. 2024;**23**(Suppl. 4):299. DOI: 10.1186/s12911-023-02375-1

[32] Awodele O, Akinyede A, Adeyemi OA, Awodele DF. Pharmacovigilance amongst doctors in private hospitals in Lagos west Senatorial District, Nigeria. The International Journal of Risk & Safety in Medicine. 2011;**23**(4):217-226. DOI: 10.3233/JRS-2011-0541

[33] Montastruc F, Taillefer de Laportaliere T. Drug-induced psychiatric disorders: A pharmacovigilance update. Therapie. 2024;**79**(2):173-179. DOI: 10.1016/j.therap.2023.09.007

[34] SchutteT,TichelaarJ,ReumermanMO, van Eekeren R, Rissmann R, Kramers C, et al. Education Committee/Working Group Research in Education of the Dutch Society of Clinical Pharmacology and Biopharmacy (NVKF&B), Utrecht, the Netherlands. Pharmacovigilance skills, knowledge and attitudes in our future doctors—A Nationwide study in the Netherlands. Basic & Clinical Pharmacology & Toxicology. 2017;**120**(5):475-481. DOI: 10.1111/bcpt.12712

[35] Hadi MA, Neoh CF, Zin RM, Elrggal ME, Cheema E. Pharmacovigilance: Pharmacists' perspective on spontaneous adverse drug reaction reporting. Integrated Pharmacy Research and Practice. 2017;**22**(6):91-98. DOI: 10.2147/IPRP.S105881

[36] Alshayban D, Mahmoud MA, Islam MA, Alshammari S, Alsulaiman D. Pharmacovigilance perception and knowledge among pharmacists and interns in Saudi Arabia. Risk Management and Healthcare Policy. 2020;**24**(13):55-61. DOI: 10.2147/RMHP.S241265

[37] Glamočlija U, Tubić B, Kondža M, Zolak A, Grubiša N. Adverse drug reaction reporting and development of pharmacovigilance systems in Bosnia and Herzegovina, Croatia, Serbia, and Montenegro: A retrospective pharmacoepidemiological study. Croatian Medical Journal. 2018;**59**(3):124-131. DOI: 10.3325/cmj.2018.59.124

[38] Tomić S, Filipović Sucić A, Plazonić A, Truban Zulj R, Macolić Sarinić V, Cudina B, et al. Regulating medicines in Croatia: Five-year experience of agency for medicinal products and medical devices. Croatian Medical Journal. 2010;**51**(2):104-112. DOI: 10.3325/cmj.2010.51.104

[39] HALMED. Farmakovigilancija. [Internet]. 2024. Available from: https://www.halmed.hr/Farmakovigilancija/Kako-prijaviti-nuspojavu/Postupak/ [Accessed: May 21, 2024]

[40] ALIMS. Farmakovigilansa. [Internet]. 2024. Available from: https://www.alims.gov.rs/ [Accessed: May 22, 2024]

[41] CINMED. Farmakovigilansa. [Internet]. 2024. Available from: https://cinmed.me/en/pharmacovigilance/adverse-reactions-to-medicines-reporting/ [Accessed: May 21, 2024]

[42] ALMBIH. Farmakovigilancija [Internet]. 2024. Available from: https://almbih.gov.ba/ [Accessed: May 22, 2024]

[43] WHO-UMC. Members [Internet]. 2024. Available from: https://who-umc.org/about-the-who-programme-for-international-drug-monitoring/member-countries/ [Accessed: May 23, 2024]

[44] Peyvandi F, Garagiola I, Mannucci PM. Post-authorization pharmacovigilance for hemophilia in Europe and the USA: Independence and transparency are keys. Blood Reviews. 2021;**49**:100828. DOI: 10.1016/j.blre.2021.100828

[45] ALMBIH. Izvještaj [Internet]. 2024. Available from: https://almbih.gov.ba/2023/01/23/izvjestaj-o-prijavama-reakcija-na-lijekove-i-cjepiva-vakcine-u-bosni-i-hercegovini-za-2022-godinu/ [Accessed: June 14, 2024]

[46] Čatić T, Begović B. The attitudes of pharmacists and physicians in Bosnia and Herzegovina towards adverse drug reaction reporting. Journal of Health Science. 2016;**6**(1):37-45. DOI: 10.17532/jhsci.2016.327

[47] Amrain M, Bečić F. Knowledge, perception, practices and barriers of healthcare professionals in Bosnia and Herzegovina towards adverse drug reaction reporting. Journal of Health Science. 2014;**4**(2):120-125. DOI: 10.17532/jhsci.2014.183

[48] Inácio P, Cavaco A, Airaksinen M. The value of patient reporting to the pharmacovigilance system: A systematic review. British Journal of Clinical Pharmacology. 2017;**83**(2):227-246. DOI: 10.1111/bcp.13098

[49] Adopo D, Daynes P, Benkebil M, Debs A, Jonville-Berra AP, Polard E, et al. Patient involvement in pharmacovigilance: Determinants and evolution of reporting from 2011 to 2020 in France. European Journal of Clinical Pharmacology. 2023;**79**(2):229-236. DOI: 10.1007/s00228-022-03422-y

[50] Prakash J, Joshi K, Malik D, Mishra O, Sachan A, Kumar B, et al. "ADR PvPI" android mobile app: Report adverse drug reaction at any time anywhere in India. Indian Journal of Pharmacology. 2019;**51**(4):236-242. DOI: 10.4103/ijp.IJP_595_18

[51] Parracha ER, Advinha AM, Lopes MJ, Oliveira-Martins S. Mobile apps for quick adverse drug reaction report: A scoping review. Pharmacoepidemiology and Drug Safety. 2023;**32**(1):19-27. DOI: 10.1002/pds.5542

Section 3

Quality Checks and Post-Market Surveillance

Chapter 6

Mitigating Challenges in Pharmacovigilance

Princy Louis Palatty, Dhanya Sacheendran and Mamatha Jayachandran

Abstract

Although pharmacovigilance is a concept well acknowledged, the practice of reporting falls short. A qualitative analysis of the challenges in pharmacovigilance revealed diverse factors contributing to the lack in reporting. Health care professionals (HCP) need to contend with their own myths and fallacies to surmount the paucity of ADR reporting. Clinical trials have standard protocols for identifying adverse events (AEs) and regulatory guidelines mandate timely reporting of ADRs, AEs, and serious adverse events (SAEs). But, in clinical practice it is trickier to obtain ADR data. Trials have active monitoring, while clinical practice relies on passive reporting from healthcare providers and patients who lack knowledge in connecting symptoms to treatment. This inadvertently leads to under-reporting of AEs and hinders the motto of patient safety. Effective pharmacovigilance hinges on skilled personnel, advanced analytical tools, data management systems, and technology. Extracting meaningful safety signals requires sophisticated data mining techniques and artificial intelligence. The vast amount of electronic health data is equally an opportunity as well as a challenge. Inconsistent reporting formats across countries could potentially lead to inaccurate or misleading interpretations. Embracing new technologies for data analysis and addressing various challenges can help in upholding patient safety in an ever-evolving healthcare landscape.

Keywords: pharmacovigilance, challenges, mitigation, reporting, adverse drug reaction (ADR) reporting, signal detection, pharmacovigilance audit

1. Introduction

Medication is a game-changer in chronic illness. Being aware that there is a drug for one's illness bestows one with confidence to live with it. Understanding your condition, managing your lifestyle, and having a strong support system are key to survival. Drugs have been the mainstay for treating most illnesses. The role of drugs is crucial in surgery such as anesthesia to keep a patient comfortable, antibiotics to ward off infections, and immunosuppressants (for transplants) to prevent graft rejection. Pre-operative medications manage anxiety, blood pressure, and more. Medications serve as a powerful tool in disease prevention, treatment, and management. In addition to the therapeutic benefits, they also pose a potential risk for unintended consequences.

Pharmacovigilance (PV) serves as a scientific discipline that embodies a systematic approach to continuously monitor and assess drug safety profiles. Vigilance surveillance is prompted to circumvent such problems. The role of vigilance is not only to look for reactions, but also prevent it. Drugs used wrongly as in medication errors (ME) could trigger adverse reactions. There has been an increased perception of the responsibility that rests on every healthcare professional to adequately report any adverse drug reaction (ADR) that may arise during clinical encounters. When a new drug is successfully marketed after undergoing clinical trials, the data generated should conceivably be able to reflect the drug's safety and efficacy. But clinical trials are conducted in carefully chosen populations and only the most common and probable adverse drug reactions are tracked [1]. However, the ADRs that occur after prolonged periods in certain specific or susceptible individuals remain unexposed. This could be attributed to an individual's genotype. When the benefits outweigh the potential risks, a drug is deemed to be relatively safe.

Monitoring the safety of medications is mandatory as it helps to keep a check in minimizing the toxicity of medications. Pharmacovigilance encompasses the complete study of drug-related adverse events. The etymology of the term pharmacovigilance is Latin and is an amalgamation of "Pharmakon" meaning "Drug" and "Vigilaire" meaning "To keep watch" [2]. The world has witnessed many disturbing events due to the administration of drugs, which have altered the course of medication safety and put into place stringent laws for the ethical conduct of clinical trials and research.

The conception of pharmacovigilance was a recent event that has evolved rapidly over the past 20 years. The WHO Program for International Drug Monitoring (WHOPIDM) was launched in 1968 with 10 member countries. This WHOPIDM gradually evolved into the WHO Pharmacovigilance Program in the mid 1970's. Now, 176 countries and territories are a part of this ambitious global initiative as of April 2023 (VIDE **Figure 1**) [3]. Its progress has given rise to a multitude of other core disciplines in the field of research and development. The World Health Organization (WHO) defines pharmacovigilance as the science and activities related to the detection, assessment, understanding, and prevention of adverse effects or other possible drug-related problem, particularly long-term and short-term adverse effects of medicines. The reporting of ADRs is steadily becoming more common and is now a legal requisite in many countries [1, 4].

Pharmacovigilance serves as a cornerstone in safeguarding medication safety throughout a drug's life cycle. The core functions of Pharmacovigilance are comprehensive Adverse Event (AE) detection and identification, signal management, Risk-Benefit profile assessment, proactive Risk Management Strategy implementation, dissemination of safety information, updating of medication safety knowledge database, and empowerment of safe and effective medication use. This discipline encompasses a collaborative effort involving various stakeholders, including pharmaceutical companies, regulatory bodies, healthcare professionals, and patients. Each of them plays a vital role in ensuring the safe and effective use of medications.

Pharmacovigilance aids in providing evidence-based information pertaining to drug-related problems (DRPs) and safety and efficacy of medications eventually helping drug regulatory authorities to formulate drug policies and various public health programs. Of the 195 recognized countries across the world, only 123 were part of the pharmacovigilance initiative as of 2016 [5]. Only recently have 47 more countries joined this venture. Lack of knowledge and sensitization regarding the importance of ADR reporting remains the major challenge in this digital era. Lack

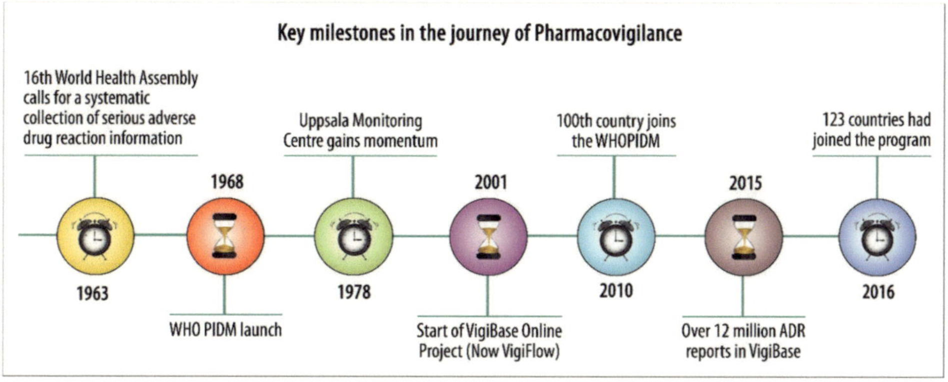

Figure 1.
Key milestones in the journey of pharmacovigilance.

of human resources and expertise, financial barriers, underreporting of ADRs, self-medication, existence of counterfeit medicines, dearth of timely documentations, and wide use of herbal and integrated medications pose further challenges in strengthening pharmacovigilance [6].

A systematic review pertaining to studies in pharmacovigilance has shed light on the fact that the disparities in PV systems in developing countries are shaped by local contextual factors such as healthcare expenditure, disease types, and political climate. These differences can result in variations in medication use and the profile of adverse effects suffered by patients, underscoring the necessity for each country to develop its own PV system [7].

Clinical assessment is crucial for precise diagnosis, necessary interventions, exploring alternative explanations, and evaluating causality. Medical expertise categorizes cases and identifies safety signals. International guidelines stress comprehensive clinical evaluation, especially for severe adverse events. Uncertainty in classifying adverse events from non-clinical trial sources hinders reporting decisions. Standardized tools, training, and technology improve analysis and classification. Educating professionals on standardized definitions promotes consistency. Signal detection identifies potential safety concerns using any available data. Standardized case evaluation protocols and training maximize data quality. Individual Case Safety Reports should adhere to a standardized format and provide concise information. The QPPV plays a crucial role in ensuring medication safety post-market release by supervising the pharmacovigilance system, establishing reporting mechanisms, analyzing ADR data, and ensuring regulatory compliance. A worldwide pharmacovigilance audit is essential for ensuring the quality and effectiveness of medication safety monitoring systems. This assessment evaluates a company's system against local and international regulations [8].

2. Good case management in pharmacovigilance

Clinical evaluation is essential to ensure accurate diagnosis, confirm necessary interventions are provided, consider alternative explanations for adverse events, and assess causality. Medical judgment is critical for case categorization and early detection of safety signals. The International Council for Harmonization (ICH) guidelines emphasize thorough clinical evaluation, especially for serious or unlisted adverse events. This helps understand the nature of events, their potential mechanism, and significance in patient safety. Effective and quality reporting is the need of the hour, and it is determined by five key elements [6, 8].

1. Valid Case Reports: Confirmed identities (patient and reporter) strengthen report reliability.

2. Defining "Seriousness": Standardized criteria for disability/incapacity ensure consistent assessment.

3. "Expectedness": Compare to existing safety information to identify potential new risks.

4. Rational Follow-up: Seek additional details to refine understanding of the event, while respecting patient privacy.

5. Clear Case Narratives: Concise, factual reports using a standardized format facilitate analysis.

There has always been an uncertainty surrounding the categorization (serious/non-serious, expected/unexpected) of adverse events (AEs) from non-clinical trial sources. This ambiguity can impede timely and appropriate reporting decisions. Standardized reporting tools, healthcare professional training, and leveraging technology can improve analysis and categorization. Enhancing healthcare professional education on standardized definitions for "seriousness" and "expectedness" fosters consistency in AE categorization across diverse reporting sources. Distinguishing between suspected ADRs and incidental events is quintessential.

Spontaneous reporting systems, designed for new safety signal detection, can be flooded with irrelevant reports. Signal detection is the process of looking for and/or identifying potential safety concerns associated with medications using data from any source. To maximize the "signal-to-noise ratio," standardized case evaluation protocols and reporter training can improve data quality. Individual Case Safety Reports (ICSRs) serve as the foundation for informed decision-making. ICSRs should follow a standardized format and must be concise. Emphasis should be placed on factual reporting of the AE, including relevant medical history, timeline of events, and any interventions implemented. Additionally, data mining techniques can objectively identify true safety signals within the reported events. Medical judgment remains paramount in converting an incidental finding to a suspected ADR [8].

To ensure proper classification and specificity of ADR terms, ideally three conditions should be fulfilled:

- case reports must be sufficiently well documented

- there must be no ambiguity regarding the nature, severity and outcome of the event

- there must be no ambiguity regarding the section(s) in the Reference Safety Information (RSI) where the appropriate information is placed.

2.1 The international council for harmonization (ICH)

The International Council for Harmonization (ICH) and individual regulatory agencies mandate that any reported case must include:

- An identifiable reporter
- An identifiable patient
- A description of the reaction/event
- A suspected medicinal product

A universally agreed-upon definition for "identifiable" reporters and patients is still lacking. This ambiguity can lead to inconsistencies in reporting practices and hinder efforts in:

- *Verifying Case Validity:* Without a clear understanding of "identifiable," it can be difficult to definitively confirm the involvement of real people in the reported ADR. This raises concerns about the overall validity and reliability of the data.
- *Preventing Duplicate Reporting:* Potential duplicate reports stemming from the same patient across different sources can occur. This redundancy can dilute the signal-to-noise ratio, obscuring genuine safety concerns.

2.2 The QPPV: champion for medication safety in pharmacovigilance

The Qualified Person Responsible for Pharmacovigilance (QPPV) is an essential figure ensuring medication safety after its market release. Within pharmacovigilance, the science of monitoring drug safety, the QPPV oversees the entire system. This includes establishing reporting processes, analyzing ADR data, and ensuring regulatory compliance. By leading risk management efforts and implementing risk reduction measures, the QPPV plays a critical role in safeguarding patients and promoting medication safety [8].

2.3 Global pharmacovigilance audit

In the realm of pharmacovigilance, the science of post-marketing drug safety, a global pharmacovigilance audit serves as a cornerstone for guaranteeing the quality and efficacy of medication safety monitoring systems. This comprehensive and independent evaluation, conducted across all geographical regions where a pharmaceutical company operates, meticulously assesses the company's pharmacovigilance system against national and international regulations [6, 8].

2.3.1 Objectives of global pharmacovigilance audit

Global pharmacovigilance audits are driven by a set of well-defined objectives:

- *Regulatory Compliance Verification:* Audits confirm the company's compliance to International Council for Harmonization (ICH) and pharmacovigilance guidelines and regional regulations.

- *Systemic Gap Identification:* Identification of potential gaps in the pharmacovigilance system allows for continuous optimization of safety monitoring practices.

- *Enhanced System Effectiveness:* Audits contribute to a more robust pharmacovigilance infrastructure in evaluating the system's effectiveness in detecting and managing potential drug safety risks.

2.3.2 Components of global pharmacovigilance audit

A global pharmacovigilance audit delves into all aspects of the company's pharmacovigilance system, encompassing a meticulous examination of:

- *Adverse Drug Reaction (ADR) Management:* Scrutiny in identifying, collecting, and meticulously recording ADRs. Also includes capturing of potential safety signals.

- *ADR Evaluation:* Assessment of severity and causality of reported ADRs with a comprehensive understanding of the potential risks associated with a medication.

- *Regulatory Reporting:* Timely reporting of ADRs to the relevant regulatory authorities verifies that a company has complied with the established protocols of ADR reporting.

- *Documentation Management:* Auditing ensures proper maintenance of all pharmacovigilance documents and safeguards the integrity of all the data.

- *Risk Management Planning (RMP):* Risk management ensures that the known benefits of a drug outweigh the potential risks for patients. This document outlines the drug's safety profile, identifying potential risks and uncertainties. It also details pharmacovigilance activities planned to gather more safety data. RMPs are required for marketing authorization applications.

2.3.3 Audit conduct: Internal expertise or external scrutiny?

The responsibility of conducting a global pharmacovigilance audit can be assigned to either internal auditors, who are members of the company's staff, or external auditors like pharmacovigilance consultants, or inspectors from regulatory agencies, who are independent and have no connection to the company's operations.

- *Internal Audits:* Internal auditors use company-specific knowledge while evaluating data. A risk of potential bias towards the existing company policies may influence the auditing process.

- *External Audits:* External auditors confer an objective perspective. They may require additional time to gain an in-depth understanding of a company's workflow process [8].

2.3.4 Benefits and challenges of pharmacovigilance audit: A balancing act

Global pharmacovigilance audits offer a multitude of benefits. Audits promote early identification and mitigation of potential drug safety risks, thus assuring efficient pharmacovigilance system functioning. It enhances the company's compliance with evolving regulations and helps foster a culture of drug safety for both pharmaceutical companies and public health.

However, no benefit presents without a challenge. Maintaining consistent audit practices across diverse geographical regions with varying regulations and infrastructure can turn out to be complex. Striking a balance between conducting a thorough audit and minimizing the burden on company resources is crucial.

Striking a balance between the benefits and challenges of conducting a pharmacovigilance audit is vital and demands significant expertise and resources. Ultimately, global pharmacovigilance audits contribute to a shared commitment—safeguarding public health through the meticulous monitoring and management of medication safety on a worldwide scale.

3. The enduring significance of the Erice declaration in pharmacovigilance

A landmark achievement, The Erice Declaration, was promulgated in 1997 following an international conference on pharmacovigilance communication. It vocalized a comprehensive vision to foster a global culture of meticulous and ethically responsible reporting of drug safety information thus ensuring medication safety.

The Declaration emphasizes collective responsibility, compelling all stakeholders to collaboratively pursue the highest ethical, professional, and scientific standards. This approach ensures that all parties involved prioritize the safety and well-being of patients throughout the medication lifecycle, from research and development to post-marketing surveillance [9]. The stakeholders involved within the pharmaceutical ecosystem include public health agencies, healthcare professionals, the pharmaceutical industry, regulatory bodies, the media, and consumers.

A salient feature of the Erice Declaration is its focus on transparent communication. It asserts the critical role that governments and policymakers play in ensuring that the information disseminated to the public concerning medications is accurate and unbiased. This empowers patients to make informed decisions about their treatment options, strengthening trust in the healthcare system and promoting medication compliance.

The Erice Declaration's principles remain highly relevant in today's ever-evolving pharmaceutical landscape [10]. As new medications are continually developed, and our understanding of existing drugs is being refined, the need for a resilient and transparent pharmacovigilance system is of paramount importance. The Declaration serves as a beacon, reminding us of the shared responsibility we all hold in safeguarding public health through open communication and collaborative efforts.

3.1 Challenges to implementing the Erice declaration in pharmacovigilance

Translating the principles of the Erice Declaration into practice necessitates a nuanced approach to navigate the complexities of information dissemination.

3.1.1 Challenge 1: Balancing transparency with public anxiety

Balancing transparency and public anxiety are significant hurdles. Disclosing potentially conflicting data, particularly in connection to vaccines, can jeopardize public health efforts by triggering a decline in immunization rates. However, withholding information regarding adverse events can erode public trust and cripple the right to informed decision-making [11].

3.1.1.1 Addressing the challenge: A multi-pronged approach

The remedy lies in communicating clear, concise, and factual data along with their risk profiles. It simplifies the interpretation of the evaluation process by openly explaining how data are assessed, and decisions are made.

3.1.2 Challenge 2: Restricted communication within regulatory systems

Fragmented communication and inefficient information exchange between national drug regulatory authorities and pharmacovigilance centers can impede effective risk management. A delay in sharing information with global counterparts can exacerbate public anxiety in the wake of potential safety concerns.

3.1.2.1 Addressing the challenge: Fostering collaboration

The challenge can be combated by the establishment of efficient communication channels and standardized reporting procedures. Timely dissemination of information with potential global implications empowers international regulators to work towards mitigating unnecessary public panic.

4. Hurdles and challenges

A Risk Management Plan (RMP) is a cornerstone document in pharmacovigilance that serves to safeguard patient safety throughout a drug's lifecycle [6, 8]. Risk Management Strategies in pharmacovigilance help in ensuring patient safety by actively monitoring the safety profile of medications aftermarket authorization. This process involves the identification, assessment, understanding, and prevention of adverse drug reactions (ADRs). To effectively manage the inherent risks associated with medications, pharmacovigilance utilizes a multi-pronged approach:

- Risk Acceptance: This strategy recognizes that no medication is entirely devoid of risks. However, a well-defined risk–benefit balance is established, where the therapeutic advantages of the medication outweigh the potential for ADRs. This is often observed in medications used to treat life-threatening conditions, where the benefits significantly outweigh the manageable risks.

- *Risk Transference:* This method involves shifting the financial responsibility associated with potential ADRs to another entity, such as an insurance company. Pharmaceutical companies may utilize insurance to mitigate the expenses related to lawsuits or compensation claims arising from severe adverse reactions.

- *Risk Avoidance:* It is a strategy employed in pharmacovigilance, involving the complete withdrawal of a medication from the market if the identified risks, especially those related to severe or life-threatening ADRs, are deemed unacceptable. This option is considered a last resort and is typically implemented after a thorough risk–benefit analysis reveals a negative balance.

- *Risk Reduction:* This is the most utilized strategy in pharmacovigilance. It focuses on actively reducing the likelihood of ADRs. Risk reduction measures encompass a variety of techniques, including dose optimization, limitations on treatment duration, refinement of patient selection criteria, and the development and implementation of new safety measures.

Establishing and maintaining a robust pharmacovigilance program comes with various obstacles that need to be addressed adequately. These could be related to the functioning model, infrastructure, and disparities between the financial aid that is needed and those that are meted out (VIDE **Figure 2**) [4].

4.1 Workforce hurdle

Pharmacovigilance systems have been in place in developed countries and in most of the developing countries. However, the efficient reporting and management of the reported ADRs is far less due to insufficient human resources. Pharmacovigilance is a meticulous process that requires groundwork activities like data collection, sensitization, and timely signal detection [11, 12].

Achieving these goals requires trained individuals capable of handling the above processes. Hence, optimal training and utilization of the available workforce to skillfully run the program is essential. To monitor the smooth workflow of the PV system, the hiring of highly qualified and trained healthcare professionals and staff is required.

4.1.1 Trust issues

Clinicians find it an affront to their ego to report ADRs, as it would be equivalent to admitting their incompetence. ADR report is not a document of evidence, though clinicians think otherwise. Such a myth must be broken. Instilling confidence in the clinicians and nurses is a priority. Reporting is the responsibility of every staff member and is the need of the hour. A “No Blame, No Shame” attitude should be employed as an organizational culture. Once this is initiated, the attitude will gain momentum.

4.1.2 Reporting incentives

The departments and the personnel reporting the most ADRs need to be acknowledged. This will help in changing the perception of others and inspire them to uphold the cause.

4.2 Financial obstacles

Running of PV systems mandates a huge financial investment. Funding of such programs is usually backed by national and state governments of a country,

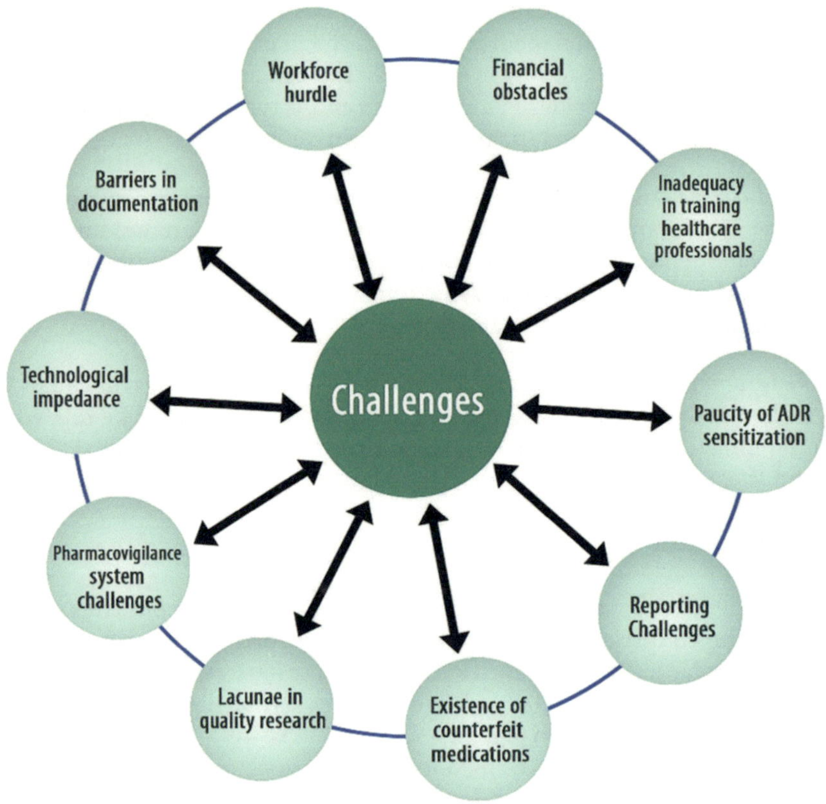
Workforce hurdle
Financial obstacles
Barriers in documentation
Inadequacy in training healthcare professionals
Technological impedance
Challenges
Paucity of ADR sensitization
Pharmacovigilance system challenges
Reporting Challenges
Lacunae in quality research
Existence of counterfeit medications

Figure 2.
Challenges to the efficient implementation of pharmacovigilance.

pharmaceutical industries, non-governmental organizations (NGO), and international organizations. Developed countries, being financially robust, can meet their needs. But investors shy from supporting such projects in developing countries primarily due to the lack of knowledge about the importance of such programs [3].

4.3 Inadequacy in training healthcare professionals

The concept of pharmacovigilance has been given due importance in health sciences curriculum. This has led to misconceptions about the responsibilities regarding who should report ADRs, the process of reporting, the appropriate time of notifying authorities, doubts regarding reporting of ADRs that are already established, and ADRs following the concomitant use of alternative systems of medications. Training programs as well as short-term courses in pharmacovigilance can be introduced at both undergraduate and postgraduate levels.

Capacity Building through eLearning: Online training modules and educational resources can provide cost-effective training, transcending geographical barriers to provide opportunities for HCPs in developing countries. Teleconferencing and online collaboration tools can connect PV program personnel in developing countries with experts in developed nations. This facilitates knowledge transfer, mentorship, and real-time support [13, 14].

4.4 Paucity of ADR sensitization

Emphasis must be laid on the fact that reporting ADRs is a social responsibility. Most ADRs go unreported because the public is unaware of their implications and that there is an option for the patient and the public to report ADRs by themselves. Public commitment can be ensured by sensitizing them through frequent awareness programs; distributing brochures, pamphlets, and relevant materials; and the use of social networking sites to promote educational videos [3, 5].

4.4.1 Broader safety concerns

Drug safety is closely linked to the patterns of drug use within society. Problems arising from irrational drug use, drug overdose, drug interactions due to polypharmacy, increasing use of alternative systems of medicine (traditional and herbal medicines), illegal sale of medicines and drugs of abuse over the internet, self-medication practices, and medication errors fall within the domain of pharmacovigilance. Monitoring systems need to become more stringent and need to evolve to address this broad scope adequately [3, 5, 15].

4.5 Reporting challenges

Suspected ADR reporting, minimizing medication errors, and ensuring medication safety is the core of PV system. Underreporting of ADRs could be due to the lack of sufficient knowledge about their implications. The hierarchy in the healthcare sector could make it difficult for individuals from lower tiers to point and report medication errors. Ensuring confidentiality of the reporting person and absence of any legal scrutiny should be emphasized during the sensitization process [3, 15].

4.5.1 Unexpected adverse reactions in pharmacovigilance

The concept of "unexpectedness" plays a crucial role in identifying potential safety signals associated with medications. Unexpectedness in pharmacovigilance is defined by regulatory guidelines. An adverse reaction is unexpected if it's absent from the drug's reference safety information (RSI), regardless of being a known medical occurrence for the treated disease. RSI documents vary depending on the drug's stage (clinical trials vs. marketed): Investigator's Brochure (DCSI section), company's core safety information, or official local data sheet (e.g., Package Insert, SPC). This distinction helps identify potential safety signals for further investigation [8].

4.5.2 Safeguarding privacy and confidentiality of data

The aspects of privacy, anonymity, and confidentiality carry great significance in pharmacovigilance. It is imperative to effectively address issues pertaining to stigma, sensitive or personal matters, and information. Anticipating and proactively dealing with the potential breach of confidentiality and anonymity is of utmost importance. Furthermore, it is crucial to ensure the preservation of privacy during the collection of data.

These privacy and confidentiality issues can be addressed by separating collected data from standard access within the healthcare system by employing alternative data storage methods. Ensure that if an electronic database is utilized, access is controlled using codes and passwords. Restrict the individuals who can access the data and anonymize the data by delinking any identifying information.

4.6 Responsibility of pharmaceutical industries

Conflicting interests within the pharmaceutical industry when dealing with drug safety issues is a major public health concern. The industry needs to prioritize patient safety and be transparent in reporting adverse drug reactions during clinical trials and post-marketing surveillance. Hesitancy to report such ADRs should be curbed by taking legal action against the offenders. The onus of responsibility lies with the regulatory authorities to lay down the necessary guidelines and policy decisions [15, 16].

4.7 Existence of counterfeit medications

Provision of good quality medicines should be ensured to keep a check on the safety profile of a drug. Unauthorized entry of counterfeit medicines into the market and the added menace of dispensing over-the-counter medications weighs down on the regulatory authorities in curbing this issue. Frequent inspections of the pharmaceutical manufacturing units and pharmacy outlets should be held with stringent actions against the offenders. The public should be made aware of the dangers of using unregistered and counterfeit medications. Healthcare professionals and pharmacists should be encouraged to report any suspected counterfeit medications [3, 16, 17].

4.8 Web-based sales and information

Uncontrolled sale of medicines across national borders has become an increasing global threat with the escalated use of web-based drug sales. Drug information in all forms and with varying levels of accuracy is made readily available across various social media platforms. Distribution of unregistered medicines, highly controlled substances, and traditional and herbal medicines with questionable safety, efficacy, and quality is rampant. This inadvertently compromises patient health as well as the purpose of pharmacovigilance [16, 17].

4.9 Lacunae in quality research

Research activities in the arena of pharmacovigilance are rudimentary in comparison to other fields of research. This reflects as deficiency in the availability of quality research outcomes. This hinders further evolution in this discipline [3, 5].

Resource Constraints: Limited funding and infrastructural deficiencies within research institutions hinder robust PV research programs in developing nations.

Knowledge Gap: Developing countries often lack established research expertise that is promptly available in developed countries.

4.9.1 Potential solutions

Filling the gaps in quality research involves a collective responsibility of local governments, pharmaceutical companies, and national and international organizations.

4.9.1.1 Role of stakeholders

Governmental Support: Allocation of dedicated budget towards PV research activities by the respective ministries of health and relevant policymakers can play a pivotal role in uplifting research interests. They can create favorable policies that incentivize research activity.

University-Industry Collaboration: Research institutions can actively seek grants and try establishing associations with pharmaceutical companies. These partnerships can provide much-needed funding and industry-relevant research focus.

4.9.1.2 International collaboration

Knowledge Transfer: Collaborative research projects involving expertise and resources from developed countries can aid knowledge transfer and impactful research.

Funding Opportunities: International funds can be leveraged for joint research ventures by engaging researchers from developed countries [3, 5].

4.9.1.3 Strategic research focus

Locally Driven Research: Research agendas can be curated depending upon landscape-specific pharmacovigilance needs and challenges. This may have a direct impact and meet the requirements of the indigenous population.

4.9.1.4 Long-term investment

Capacity Building: Investing in training programs is essential for nurturing sustainable research infrastructure and fostering a tradition of knowledge creation. This can pave way as a comprehensive strategy in tackling research gaps and enhancing valuable global contributions in pharmacovigilance. This will address pressing challenges and enrich the global knowledge base for the benefit of all stakeholders.

4.10 Bridging the pharmacovigilance gap: a strategic approach for developing countries

Developing countries often face significant challenges in implementing pharmacovigilance (PV) programs [18–20].

4.10.1 Current landscape

Limited or Absent Systems: Many developing countries do not have established national PV systems. Hence the systematic monitoring of medication safety is compromised.

Resource Constraints: Lack of international tie-ups, insufficient staffing, and limited geographical reach take a toll on the proper functioning of the existing PV systems.

Scope Inadequacy: Traditional systems of herbal medications, self-medication practices, and vaccine safety are often overlooked and frequently neglected. This culminates in a deficient PV reporting system [18, 20].

4.10.1.1 Proposed solutions

National System Implementation: The World Health Organization (WHO) has laid down minimum requirements for establishing national PV systems. Developing countries should strive to adhere to and implement these standards by utilizing international aid to address resource constraints.

Capacity Building for Existing Systems: Betterment of the existing PV systems can be achieved through targeted staff training, development of infrastructure, and improved data collection and analysis processes.

Expanding the Scope of PV: A thorough understanding of medication safety necessitates herbal medications, self-medication practices, and vaccine safety to be incorporated into PV monitoring activities.

4.10.2 Promoting medication safety culture

Medication Safety Accreditation: The formulation of a national medication safety accreditation program can lead to sustained improvement in PV practices. Setting measurable standards and recognizing excellence can strengthen the culture of medication safety.

Regulatory Framework Development: The establishment of clear regulations and stringent guidelines specific to PV and medication safety will ensure effective implementation [19, 20].

These strategic approaches offer a roadmap for developing countries to bridge the current pharmacovigilance gap and create a safer medication environment for all.

4.11 Technological impedance

Pharmacovigilance (PV) is undergoing significant transformations driven by the emergence of novel digital technologies, its applications, and the influence of social media. This ensures a plethora of opportunities to significantly improve PV practices globally [3, 21].

4.11.1 Challenges and considerations

Bridging the Digital Divide: Unequal access to digital technology and innovations in developing countries is a barrier to equitable participation in ADR reporting and data analysis [3, 20, 21].

Data Privacy and Security: Data security measures to safeguard patient privacy will help to build trust and encourage more public reporting of ADRs.

4.11.2 Revolutionizing data collection and reporting

Mobile Health (mHealth) Applications: User-friendly mHealth applications can empower patients and healthcare professionals (HCPs) for convenient ADR reporting directly into PV systems. This can dramatically increase reporting rates, facilitating the real-time identification of potential safety concerns [3].

Social Media Listening: Harnessing the power of social media platforms can be used for passive data collection on medication use and detecting potential ADRs. Advanced analytics tools, relevant conversations, and emerging trends can be systematically identified and analyzed. Social media platforms can effectively disseminate clear, concise, and up-to-date medication safety information to HCPs and the public. Interactive features utilizing telemedicine and online platforms can encourage open dialog and address public concerns in a timely and transparent manner [5, 11].

Integration with the Internet of Things (IoT): The rapidly flourishing realm of the Internet of Things (IoT) offers unlimited possibilities. Advent of the revolutionary smart pill bottles and wearable medication adherence tracking devices can be channeled for possible capturing of physiological data to potentially signal adverse reactions. Integrating these data with PV systems can provide a more holistic view of medication safety [21].

4.12 Data utility

The CIOMS V Working Group recognized the critical need for clear definitions regarding "identifiable patients" in pharmacovigilance. Availability of one or more data elements like age, sex, initials, date of birth, name, or patient number would automatically qualify a patient as identifiable. Clear identification aids in confirming case validity and minimizing the risk of duplicate reporting. In the event where clear identity data are missing, reports mentioning a definite number of patients experiencing an AE (e.g., "Two patients experienced...") would be considered legitimate for initial reporting. Importance of data utility while safeguarding privacy is of paramount importance [8]. This can be achieved by these approaches.

- Individual patient data (age, sex) are preferred for better case evaluation.
- Unidentified cases can be reported as "notification letters" with clear limitations mentioned.
- Hearsay-based reports are discouraged, with priority given to credible sources.
- For serious or unexpected ADRs, reporting thresholds are lowered to capture potential safety risks even with limited identifiability.

4.13 Barriers in documentation

Documenting the PV related activities is integral to developing the necessary interventions and improving the PV practices. Lack of time and ADRs considered not serious enough by pharmacists to report were barriers to ADR reporting. Further training and education about the types of ADRs to be reported can help to improve the reporting of ADRs. The factors deterring adequate ADR reporting were identified as knowledge gaps, insufficient human resources, limited training of HCPs and PV personnel, excessive workload, poor supportive supervision, lack of quality supervisory visit, and weak implementation of Adverse Events Following Immunization (AEFI) policy guidance. Others pertinent issues included poor funding and logistics, dearth of dedicated budget provision, socio-economic and infrastructural deficits, geographical barriers, limited Information and Communication Technology (ICT) skills, poor feedback, and weak community engagement by the health workers. Facilitators of ADR reporting were identified as provision of extra time for ADR reporting, incentives, continuous medical education and training programs, reminders to report, and availability of an online ADR reporting system [5, 6, 8, 17].

The transition from paper-based to electronic pharmacovigilance (PV) systems offers significant advantages, but not without its hurdles.

4.14 Digital infrastructure issues

Limited Internet Access: Unavailability, unreliability, and high cost of internet connectivity can significantly hinder the effective use of electronic reporting systems.

4.14.1 System design and implementation challenges

Hybrid Systems: Relying on a mix of paper and electronic reporting tools can create confusion and inefficiencies. Ideally, a seamless, unified system is more efficient.

System Usability: Complex or user-unfriendly electronic systems can discourage healthcare professionals (HCPs) from utilizing them [17, 21].

4.14.2 Organizational challenges

Coordination Issues: Inadequate coordination can hamper the smooth operation and data management of the electronic system. Changes in the healthcare management structure within a country can disrupt established workflows and create delays in adapting to a new electronic reporting system [3, 5].

4.14.3 Strategies to overcome these hurdles

Mindful investment in Digital Infrastructure can help expand internet access and affordability thus enabling a user-friendly, single electronic reporting system. This can help in streamlining the PV process by eliminating existing disparities. Also, providing training and technical support to navigate the electronic system effectively will enable a smooth transition and integration of newer technologies. All these strategies facilitate clear communication and stronger co-ordination within national and international PV centers.

5. Novel ways to mitigate problems in pharmacovigilance

The field of PV is progressing, and the coming decade presents a unique confluence of significant challenges and exciting possibilities that can redefine the ideology about pharmacovigilance.

Historically, PV has primarily focused on identifying adverse drug reactions (ADRs). While ADR identification has remained the primary focus of PV, the future of PV lies in expanding our knowledge of a drug's safety profile. A comprehensive understanding of drug safety profiles interlaced with pharmacogenetics and pharmacogenomics can lead to the development of targeted interventions, potentially mitigating unforeseen risks and optimizing medication use [5, 6]. This multifaceted approach can foster the identification of previously unknown safety concerns, ultimately accelerating the development of safer medications. The last two decades have seen the concept of evidence-based medicine (EBM) gaining momentum. Evidence-based risk benefit assessments and their incorporation in decision-making has enabled greater transparency, thus improving medication safety for patients [15, 16].

A strong scientific foundation will lead to the development of more rigorous and effective PV methodologies. This can be achieved by ensuring wider accessibility to training and resources by offering dedicated robust academic programs, and encouraging collaboration between diverse disciplines, such as pharmacology, statistics, epidemiology, and various clinical departments.

The future demands the development and implementation of a standardized audit process based on established "good pharmacovigilance practice" principles. The lack of standardized audit processes for PV practices can raise concerns about quality and consistency. Standardized audits will provide a framework for ensuring the integrity and reliability of PV data. Effective comparisons and collaboration between PV programs in different countries can lead to a more unified global approach to medication safety.

5.1 One size does not fit all: strategic shifts in how to engage with countries

A "one size fits all" approach in PV engagement with different countries is impractical and ineffective. Various countries have healthcare systems with diverse levels of development, infrastructure, and reporting mechanisms for ADRs. A standardized approach might overwhelm resource-limited settings, while underestimating the needs of more developed ones. Regulations governing pharmacovigilance practices differ between countries. A one-size-fits-all strategy would not consider these variations, potentially hindering compliance and data collection efforts. Cultural attitudes towards medication use, reporting practices, and communication styles vary significantly. A sensitive and adaptable approach can overcome this [1, 6].

Risk-Based Stratification: Countries can be categorized based on their resource availability, healthcare infrastructure, and disease burden, thus allowing for targeted interventions.

Culturally Appropriate Resources: Developing culturally appropriate resource materials and training programs that resonate with the local audience would be beneficial.

Gathering Local Expertise: Partnering with local healthcare professionals and research institutions builds trust and facilitates data collection that is curated according to regional needs.

Technological Innovation: Utilizing innovative technologies like mobile health platforms and telemedicine can improve ADR reporting in resource-limited settings.

6. Sustaining pharmacovigilance during a pandemic

Historical timelines bear proof to the fact that pandemics pose a significant threat to global health, causing widespread illness and mortality. However, their impact extends far beyond the immediate effects of the infectious disease itself. Pandemics also have a profound ability to disrupt and overburden healthcare systems, hindering their capacity to deliver essential services. Pandemics lead to a rapid influx of patients seeking treatment. The healthcare sector is overwhelmingly pushed to its limits of providing critical care management. This creates staff shortages and burnout among the existing personnel, further compromising their ability to deliver services. Prioritizing care of critically ill patients remains the mainstay in dealing with a pandemic, leading to delays in essential care for other health conditions. Under such circumstances, the efficiency of extended services like pharmacovigilance activities remains questionable [21].

Off-label use of many drugs is experimented both by healthcare professionals as well as by the public. This can aggravate the incidence of drug-related adverse events (AE). Off-label use hinders proper reporting of such drug-related AEs.

6.1 Pressing issues

Globalized Landscape: Disparities in healthcare infrastructure and regulatory frameworks across countries can impede effective collaboration and data sharing. This fragmentation creates obstacles in establishing a comprehensive understanding of drug safety during a global health crisis [15].

Surge in Data: Pandemics demand rapid development and deployment of novel therapeutics, leading to a surge in ADR reporting data. Due to this heavy influx, timely identification of safety signals is compromised.

Expanding Safety Scope: Traditional PV practices primarily focus on ADRs within defined parameters. However, pandemics demand a broader perspective encompassing medication errors, self-medication practices, and potential interactions with traditional medicines [16].

Vaccine Hesitancy: The spread of misleading information and a general distrust can lead to vaccine hesitancy, hindering efforts to contain the pandemic. Low vaccination rates can prolong the pandemic and allow for the emergence of new variants, further straining healthcare systems [21].

6.2 Enhancing pharmacovigilance practices

Real-time Data Management Systems: Implementing real-time data collection and analysis platforms is essential. This allows for expedited identification of probable safety concerns and more informed decision-making.

Expanding Data Sources: Diversifying data sources beyond traditional reporting methods by mobilizing patient registries, social media platforms, and healthcare provider networks can deliver a more comprehensive picture of drug safety across global populations [16, 18, 20, 21].

Public Education Initiatives: Empowering the public with accurate and accessible information about safe medication use is important. This can reduce risks associated with self-medication practices and wrong information.

Addressing these challenges and implementing the possible solutions, PV can be significantly strengthened. This will help maintain the continued safety and efficacy of medications during a pandemic, ultimately safeguarding public health on a global scale.

7. Pharmacovigilance from a global perspective

Despite the rise in PV development and utilization in developing countries, there exists a gap in the efforts to evaluate, assess, and monitor the status, growth, and impact of their systems and activities. The WHO advises that PV systems should integrate evaluation and assessment mechanisms with defined performance criteria. Evaluation of existing conditions can aid in outlining the elements of a sustainable PV strategy and identifying areas for enhancement, laying the groundwork for improved public health and medication safety planning. Research studies have identified constraints associated with the assessment instruments employed in appraising PV efficacy [7]. Four constraints intrinsic to the Indicator-Based Pharmacovigilance Assessment Tool [IPAT], such as the absence of established sensitivity and specificity, potential inaccuracies in response quantification during scoring, dependence on respondents' self-reports, and the need for customization at the local level due to limited tool testing and validation were identified in one of the studies.

Few other studies pointed out the limitations of employing the WHO PV indicators. The issues brought to the forefront were shortage of adequately trained personnel, substandard documentation practices, and the necessity for more thorough surveys that emerging systems may struggle to conduct. The studies highlighted the absence of a scoring system within the WHO PV indicators that hindered the quantification of indices.

Effective action and long-term planning in PV can only be realized when a sustainable budget is combined with other structural elements of the system. A survey by WHO has revealed that financial support is crucial for conducting PV activities within a given context, symbolizing the commitment and political will of the sponsors. For the optimal utilization of financial resources, the investment strategies should focus on diverse country characteristics, such as size, population, and the expected reporting rate of the system [7].

Underreporting has been identified as a significant obstacle in both developing as well as developed nations. Studies have identified that all incidents are not being reported possibly due to passive reporting. This underreporting compromises collection of comprehensive data on drug safety, quality, and efficacy. This in turn impinges on the process of data analysis, signal detection, regulatory measures, and data transmission.

Identifying and rectifying the above-mentioned inconsistencies will pave the way for a better implementation of the pharmacovigilance program. The current technological era favors the utilization of artificial intelligence, which is now a key component in the PV workflow [7].

8. The artificial intelligence wave

Artificial intelligence (AI) is rapidly transforming the field of pharmacovigilance. The explosion of PV data is a goldmine for AI algorithms to analyze the huge quantum of information by automation [22]. Challenges in resource-limited settings include the absence of robust databases, inadequate human resources, underdeveloped AI technology, and lack of government support. Addressing these challenges through collaborative efforts, research initiatives, and advanced machine-learning algorithms can enhance AI-based pharmacovigilance capabilities in settings with limited resources. A comprehensive PV database is essential to fully utilize AI technology. Developed and developing nations have extensive established PV databases. Low- and middle-income countries (LMICs) on the other hand face challenges in establishing a strong database due to underreporting, inadequate infrastructure, and limited resources and policies [23]. By integrating essential data like laboratory results, medical records, and medication orders, electronic health records (EHRs) can be efficiently used for AI-based PV work process.

Limited training opportunities and financial assistance in LMICs contribute to a shortage of healthcare professionals and infrastructural development in pharmacovigilance. The emergence of AI-based pharmacovigilance poses a challenge for LMICs with limited access to AI-related training programs. Integrating PV education into healthcare training curricula and introducing specialized postgraduate courses in AI-driven PV can address this issue. Investing in education and training can help LMICs overcome the shortage of healthcare professionals for pharmacovigilance and improve patient safety. Without a sustainable budget, the long-term effectiveness of pharmacovigilance systems is at risk. China and India serve as examples where financial backing has enabled the establishment of sustainable systems [24].

There are two main obstacles that AI-based pharmacovigilance (PV) encounters in settings with limited resources: data integration and data annotation. The most significant technological challenge for AI-based PV is term variation. The terms used, such as drug and disease names, are often informal and highly variable. The description of side effects may lack clarity, and grammar and spelling mistakes may be common [25]. Furthermore, the diversity of local languages further complicates data processing, integration, and normalization. Concept normalization is a solution that helps address this issue by enhancing data quality, reducing dimensions, increasing retrieval recall, and integrating various data sources. Standardized medical vocabularies (SNOMED CT, LOINC) can turn out to be possible game changers [22]. They improve data quality, leading to more accurate and complete detection of potential side effects. This, in turn, strengthens LMIC pharmacovigilance systems and fosters international collaboration [23, 24].

Enhanced data sharing and validation through multinational collaboration streamlines data collection and enables the creation of an AI-driven pharmacovigilance platform in resource-limited settings. This allows LMICs to exchange and verify data, representing diverse regions and populations [23]. Spontaneous reports from healthcare professionals and consumers may be limited by biases and underreporting. AI algorithms have been used to identify pharmacovigilance signals from multiple data sources, such as biomedical literature, knowledge graphs, and genetic information. Combining these diverse sources provides a comprehensive view of drug safety [25].

In resource-limited settings, special populations such as women, children, and indigenous groups are often underrepresented in existing data sources. This ongoing challenge of increasing population coverage can be addressed by reactive learning algorithms that adapt to the changing landscape. Engaging various stakeholders is key to establishing a sustainable AI-driven pharmacovigilance system nationwide. The involvement of government bodies, pharmaceutical firms, technology companies, healthcare institutions, and patient advocacy organizations is crucial for a comprehensive approach [22, 25].

9. Conclusions

The field of medicine is constantly evolving with new medications getting introduced frequently. Continuous monitoring of ADR data helps in fostering a vigilant environment. By staying attuned to emerging trends, healthcare professionals can aptly identify and explore novel safety concerns. This proactive approach ensures that patient safety remains at the forefront in the healthcare sector. AI is poised to play a transformative role in the future of pharmacovigilance. Harnessing the power of AI can facilitate a more comprehensive understanding of drug safety. In essence, ADR reporting with signal detection empowers healthcare workers to act as guardians, uncovering potential threats and implementing preventive measures before they detrimentally impact patients. ADR reporting with a constant lookout for signals helps to contribute to medication safety. Preventing ADRs is only one of the benefits of pharmacovigilance. Premedication, unintended complications, and known cumulative toxicities can also be identified and prevented, when there is a constant vigil.

Author details

Princy Louis Palatty*, Dhanya Sacheendran and Mamatha Jayachandran
Department of Pharmacology, Amrita School of Medicine, Amrita Institute of Medical Sciences, Amrita Vishwa Vidyapeetham, Kochi, India

*Address all correspondence to: drprincylouispalatty@gmail.com

IntechOpen

© 2024 The Author(s). Licensee IntechOpen. This chapter is distributed under the terms of the Creative Commons Attribution License (http://creativecommons.org/licenses/by/4.0), which permits unrestricted use, distribution, and reproduction in any medium, provided the original work is properly cited.

References

[1] Beninger P. Pharmacovigilance: An overview. Clinical Therapeutics. 2018;**40**(12):1991-2004. DOI: 10.1016/j.clinthera.2018.07.012. Epub 2018 Aug 17

[2] Shuka SS, Bina G, Pandey R, Rao SP, Singh V, Amber V. Importance of pharmacovigilance in Indian pharmaceutical industry. Asian Journal of Research in Pharmaceutical Science. 2012;**2**:04-08

[3] Al-Worafi YM, Kassab YW, Alseragi WM, Almutairi MS, Ahmed A, Ming LC, et al. Pharmacovigilance and adverse drug reaction reporting: A perspective of community pharmacists and pharmacy technicians in Sana'a, Yemen. Therapeutics and Clinical Risk Management. 2017;**13**:1175-1181. DOI: 10.2147/TCRM.S140674

[4] Fornasier G, Francescon S, Leone R, Baldo P. An historical overview over pharmacovigilance. International Journal of Clinical Pharmacy. 2018;**40**(4):744-747. DOI: 10.1007/s11096-018-0657-1. Epub 2018 Jun 15

[5] Lavertu A, Vora B, Giacomini KM, Altman R, Rensi S. A new era in pharmacovigilance: Toward real-world data and digital monitoring. Clinical Pharmacology and Therapeutics. 2021;**109**(5):1197-1202. DOI: 10.1002/cpt.2172. Epub 2021 Feb 28

[6] World Health Organization (WHO). Pharmacovigilance [Internet]. 2024 [cited 2024 Apr 06]. Available from: https://www.who.int/teams/regulation-prequalification/regulation-and-safety/pharmacovigilance

[7] Garashi HY, Steinke DT, Schafheutle EI. A systematic review of pharmacovigilance systems in developing countries using the WHO pharmacovigilance indicators. Therapeutic Innovation & Regulatory Science. 2022;**56**(5):717-743. DOI: 10.1007/s43441-022-00415-y. Epub 2022 Jun 3

[8] CIOMS - Council for International Organizations of Medical Sciences. n.d. Available from: https://cioms.ch/ [Accessed: June 4, 2024]

[9] Jeetu G, Anusha G. Pharmacovigilance: A worldwide master key for drug safety monitoring. Journal of Young Pharmacists. 2010;**2**(3):315-320. DOI: 10.4103/0975-1483.66802

[10] Hugman B. The Erice declaration: The critical role of communication in drug safety. Drug Safety. 2006;**29**(1): 91-93. DOI: 10.2165/00002018-200629010-00007

[11] Palaian S. Chapter 9 - Pharmacovigilance Practices and Activities: Issues, Challenges, and Future Direction, Social and Administrative Aspects of Pharmacy in Low- and Middle-Income Countries. Elsevier Science and Technology, Academic Press; 2018. pp. 145-162. ISBN 9780128112281. DOI: 10.1016/B978-0-12-811228-1.00009-1

[12] Moore N, Berdaï D, Blin P, Droz C. Pharmacovigilance - The next chapter. Thérapie. 2019;**74**(6):557-567. DOI: 10.1016/j.therap.2019.09.004. Epub 2019 Oct 1

[13] Bihan K, Lebrun-Vignes B, Funck-Brentano C, Salem JE. Uses of pharmacovigilance databases: An overview. Thérapie. 2020;**75**(6):591-598. DOI: 10.1016/j.therap.2020.02.022. Epub 2020 Feb 26

[14] Lewis DJ, McCallum JF. Utilizing advanced technologies to augment pharmacovigilance systems: Challenges and opportunities. Therapeutic Innovation & Regulatory Science. 2020;**54**(4):888-899. DOI: 10.1007/s43441-019-00023-3. Epub 2019 Dec 28

[15] Dikshit RK. Challenges in pharmacovigilance. Indian Journal of Pharmacology. 2010;**42**(6):333. DOI: 10.4103/0253-7613.71882

[16] Trifirò G, Crisafulli S. A new era of pharmacovigilance: Future challenges and opportunities. Frontiers in Drug Safety and Regulation. 2022;**2**. DOI: 10.3389/fdsfr.2022.866898

[17] Li Y, Wu Y, Jiang T, Xing H, Xu J, Li C, et al. Opportunities and challenges of pharmacovigilance in special populations: A narrative review of the literature. Therapeutic Advances in Drug Safety. 2023;**14**:20420986231200746. DOI: 10.1177/20420986231200746

[18] Stegmann JU, Jusot V, Menang O, Gardiner G, Vesce S, Volpe S, et al. Challenges and lessons learned from four years of planning and implementing pharmacovigilance enhancement in sub-Saharan Africa. BMC Public Health. 2022;**22**(1):1568. DOI: 10.1186/s12889-022-13867-6

[19] Desai M. Pharmacovigilance and spontaneous adverse drug reaction reporting: Challenges and opportunities. Perspectives in Clinical Research. 2022;**13**(4):177-179. DOI: 10.4103/picr.picr_169_22. Epub 2022 Sep 27

[20] Wong J, Prieto-Alhambra D, Rijnbeek PR, Desai RJ, Reps JM, Toh S. Applying machine learning in distributed data networks for pharmacoepidemiologic and pharmacovigilance studies: Opportunities, challenges, and considerations. Drug Safety. 2022;**45**(5):493-510. DOI: 10.1007/s40264-022-01158-3. Epub 2022 May 17

[21] Mercier N, Belhadi D, DeChanet A, Delmas C, Saillard J, Dumousseaux M, et al. Management of pharmacovigilance during the COVID-19 pandemic crisis by the safety department of an academic sponsor: Lessons learnt and challenges from the EU DisCoVeRy clinical trial. Pharmacology Research & Perspectives. 2023;**11**(3):e01072. DOI: 10.1002/prp2.1072

[22] Murali K, Kaur S, Prakash A, Medhi B. Artificial intelligence in pharmacovigilance: Practical utility. Indian Journal of Pharmacology. 2019;**51**(6):373-376. DOI: 10.4103/ijp.IJP_814_19. Epub 2020 Jan 16

[23] Babigumira JB, Stergachis A, Choi HL, Dodoo A, Nwokike J, Garrison LP Jr. A framework for assessing the economic value of pharmacovigilance in low- and middle-income countries. Drug Safety. 2014;**37**(3):127-134. DOI: 10.1007/s40264-014-0143-1

[24] Olsson S, Pal SN, Stergachis A, Couper M. Pharmacovigilance activities in 55 low- and middle-income countries: A questionnaire-based analysis. Drug Safety. 2010;**33**(8):689-703. DOI: 10.2165/11536390-000000000-00000

[25] Ventola CL. Big data and pharmacovigilance: Data mining for adverse drug events and interactions. Pharmacy and Therapeutics. 2018;**43**(6):340-351

Chapter 7

Perspective Chapter: A Narrative Review of Pharmacovigilance – Report of Adverse Drug Reactions in Mexico

Miguel Luján Estrada, Aivle Libertad Hernández Caamaño and Karla Roman Flores

Abstract

Drugs are potent and capable of modifying homeostatic mechanisms. They do not create new functions and only modify existing ones. Drugs that appeared in recent years can increase or decrease organic functions, with greater potency and selectivity than previous, although, there is no evidence to suggest that they are safer. The desirable and undesirable effects of the drugs depend on factors that are regulated by the host, the drug, and the environment. Mexico (126 million inhabitants) should generate at least 25,200 useful notifications of Adverse Drug Reactions (ADR) each year. This goal had not been achieved until recently, due to the bad quality of the reports and to the lack of feedback to the reporters. Physicians encounter challenges in reporting: (a) access to an efficient reporting mechanism; (b) knowledge of what and how to report an ADR: fear of Punitive or Legal Ramifications. (c) Lack of Instruction During Training; (d) Excessive Paperwork and Time Constraints; (e) Incentive Gap: The absence of incentives for reporting ADRs contribute to lack of reporting. State shall record and communicate to the physicians all suspected adverse reaction that accomplishes the sufficient quality of the information to reduce the underreporting.

Keywords: drugs, adverse drug reactions, reporting, underreporting, Mexico

1. Introduction

The ability to predict the occurrence of an adverse effect depends on part on the frequency of use of the drug. This makes it possible to foretell, in many cases, the presence of some adverse events that have a high incidence of occurrence, such as nausea that occurs with the use of some non-steroidal antipyretic analgesics, or vomiting induced by the administration of opioids. However, there are drugs that can induce adverse effects that occur very rarely; the observation of such adverse reactions depends on the size of the user's population and the frequency of drug use. Adverse effects have had presentations as low as 1 in 10,000, or 1 in 100,000; there are even reports of extremely rare events being observed in 1 in 1,000,000 users. However, the fact that they occur infrequently does not mean that they are without clinical significance. In fact, many of these adverse effects can lead to death or serious clinical changes. With the increase in the development of new drugs, there has been an increase in the possibility of new adverse effects, and unfortunately, these effects occur more frequently in those patients for whom the drug that produced it was inappropriately prescribed. Proper knowledge and interpretation of the adverse effects produced by a medicine, as well as their incidence, are essential for the rational use of medicines and help clinicians to make decisions about administering a medicine to a patient and to consider the potential risks that the patient faces when using the medicine to be prescribed.

The word drug is used to refer to any chemical substance that affects the biological processes of life [1]. The affected process can lead to a beneficial or harmful effect, as in the case of poisons or toxins. Drugs can cure diseases, treat symptoms, as aids in diagnosis, help for disease prevention, and to promote health; if a drug has any of these uses, it is a medicine. Although most people believe that drugs cure diseases, there are few drugs that are curative [2]; the most representative examples of curative drugs are antibiotics. Most medicines help treat the symptoms of diseases. For example, oral hypoglycemics agents, by increasing the release of insulin—which is a modification of a physiological parameter of a patient—can decrease glucose concentrations and help the patient to *control* their diabetes. There are also medications such as antiparkinsonians, which do not cure the patient but do help to reduce the most important symptoms of this disease, such as tremor. Drugs are aids in diagnosis, can mention radioactive substances, which facilitate or guide us in the diagnosis of diseases, such as cancer of the thyroid gland. On the other hand, vaccines are the drugs *par excellence*, which help us prevent diseases, and of course, there are others that help us promote good health, such as vitamins, food supplements, and contraceptives.

It should note that drugs only modify functions quantitatively, never qualitatively [1], and they are not capable of creating new functions. The presentation of adverse effects, in most cases, are only extensions of the effects produced by the medications. However, to date very few drugs are highly selective, and therefore, adequate prediction of the type of adverse effects can be difficult. In general, drugs are substances that have a multiplicity of actions, and they are "promiscuous"; that is, they interact with different sites of action, and their effect depends on the dose used, since this causes different responses by activating multiple physiological systems at high doses.

In general, most drugs are produced by the pharmaceutical industries. There are three types of pharmaceutical companies: research, generic, and high-tech [2]. The companies that are in the first group are based for their operation on the discovery and development of new drugs based on innovation, risking substantial amounts of economic resources in the search for novel products. The second group is engaged in the manufacture and sale of generic products, discovered by other companies, and commercialized when the patent for such products has already expired. They compete on price, and their efforts are aimed at price controls, not the discovery of new drugs. The third group is made up of high-tech companies, where recent technical advances are used, especially in the field of biotechnology applied to biological engineering to produce biologics such as vaccines, antibodies, and insulin [2].

However, the purpose of the industry is to make a profit. Although, the occurrence of side effects or adverse events when administering a drug cannot be discarded, still is observed that drugs are highly beneficial. There are important examples in the literature that illustrate these aspects [2]; some of them—perhaps the most representative—are related to the decrease in the number of cases of some diseases that occurred in 1940 and that were modified in 1982, where there is a difference of more than 40 years and mortality has decreased significantly. We can take diphtheria as an example: in 1940 there were 15,536 cases of diphtheria reported in the USA, and in 1982 only two cases presented, and the percentage reduction was 99.9%. For measles, in 1940 291,162 cases of measles appeared in the USA and in 1982, 1700 cases, the percentage reduction was 99.4%. In the case of poliomyelitis, 58,000 cases were observed in 1940, and eight cases were registered in 1982 [2]. The above data indicate that the percentage reduction in morbidity and mortality of diseases has been spectacular in some cases. This reduction has been the result of the development of useful vaccines and drugs against these diseases. True, these drugs have adverse effects, but the risk–benefit ratio has shifted toward the positive. This shows that the use of medications is and will continue to be critical to reducing morbidity and mortality in individuals.

The therapeutic usefulness of a drug depends mainly on its ability to produce the desired effects with only a minimum of undesirable effects; thus, one of the most important characteristics of a drug must be the selectivity of its action [1]. For this reason, we must consider that the most desired characteristics is efficacy, the ability to produce a response at therapeutic doses; on the other hand, safety is related to not producing life-threatening side effects and is that the side effects are not so bothersome for the patient that they must interrupt treatment.

Most medications are highly effective. However, they do produce adverse effects. The spectrum of undesirable effects can be broad and ill-defined. In fact, drugs produce many effects, but only one of them is considered as the main effect, and the others are considered as undesirable or side effects [3]. But before we go any further, we should ask what is an adverse reaction?

2. Definition of adverse reaction

The World Health Organization (WHO) defines an adverse reaction as "one that is harmful, unwanted, and occurs at doses used for prophylaxis, diagnosis, or therapy or for the modification of a physiological function". Another definition or an extension of this definition is "any deleterious response or change in the patient's condition that is induced by a drug and that occurs at therapeutic doses and that requires treatment, decrease, or discontinuation of drug therapy or suggests that future use of the drug by the patient poses a high risk to the patient." The latter points out that adverse reactions can occur in any study of drug administration. Drug abuse and accidental or induced poisoning are not classified as adverse drug reactions (ADRs), although they are considered within a large context of risk in the use of drugs [4]. The WHO definition does not specify whether failure of therapeutic purpose is an adverse reaction—in fact, it is currently a point of contention at the WHO—but it is referred as therapeutic failure. The reasons for treatment failure may be related to the medication or the patient. Drug-related failures can occur due to the wrong choice of drug for the therapeutic situation, errors in the prescription or administration of the drug, drug interactions, variations in bioavailability in inappropriate formulation priority, or inadequate route or route of administration [4]. Patient-related therapeutic failures occur due to poor patient adherence to the proposed therapeutic scheme, or variations in bioavailability due to transient pathological states of the patient such as diarrhea that affects absorption. ADRs frequently occur in situations where too many drugs are present, while therapeutic failures occur in situations where there is little availability of the drug. Because disease progression is often a confounding factor, treatment failure and ADRs are often difficult to differentiate. The incidence of therapeutic failure, on the other hand, is similar quantitatively to the prevalence of ADRs [3]. Studies in the USA have identified adverse drug reactions (ADRs) as between the fourth and sixth leading cause of death (higher than motor vehicle accidents, breast cancer or AIDS), with an estimated fatality rate of 0.32% among hospitalized patients. A single adverse drug event (ADE) has been costed at approximately US$2500, and hospitals in the USA pay approximately US$4 billion per year for drug-induced injuries. In another study in a nursing home, it was observed that, for every dollar spent on drugs, US$1.33 was spent on the treatment of drug-related problems [5].

3. Classification of adverse reactions

The presence of an ADR leads the physician to decide on a series of measures that are related to the type of reaction. At this point it is necessary to ask the following question: How are adverse drug reactions classified? In general, the classification is as follows [6]:

1. Intrinsic. By other authors [3], called type A reactions, this type of reactions is considered as an extension of the pharmacological effects of the drug or its metabolites. Its features are as follows:

   - Pharmacologically predictable.
   - Dose-dependent.
   - High incidence.
   - Low mortality.
   - Treatment: dose adjustment or temporary discontinuation.

It depends on the chemical properties of the drug and is usually dose dependent. Intrinsic adverse reactions can constitute 70-80% of the total of these types of events, they are predictable and therefore can be avoided in some of the cases, and when they do occur, they can sometimes be considered as iatrogenic [6].

Type A adverse reactions are due to an extension of the pharmacological actions of the drug. The intensity of the reaction is in relation to the dose of the drug administered; for this reason, the appropriate treatment for most cases includes the correct dosage adjustment [3].

An example of this type of adverse reaction is aspirin toxicity, also hypoglycemia secondary to oral hypoglycemic or drowsiness with antihistamines first generation.

2. Extrinsic. Also called type B reactions. These types of reactions are difficult to predict, less frequent, and therefore are presented only when many patients have been treated for the drug in question [6], but when they do occur, they can be extremely dangerous, as they more often cause mortality. The reactions of this group are individual-dependent, not dose-related [3], difficult to reproduce in animals, and comparatively uncommon; when any of these reactions appear, in addition to symptomatic measures, the drug should be discontinued [3]. These reactions are associated with enzyme deficiencies in the patient, such as glucose-6-phosphate dehydrogenase deficiency, which increases the vulnerability of red blood cells. Other types of reactions in this group have an

immunological basis. As hypersensitivity reactions. Drug allergies are extremely variable in their presentation and remain in the individual throughout their life. Clinical manifestations may include asthma, anaphylaxis, hemolytic anemia, hepatitis, lupus, etc. The occurrence of these manifestations may be concurrent and present at the onset or subsequent use of the drug. Why non-immunogenic small molecules can trigger allergic reactions is not well known [7].

Under normal conditions, for a molecule as generator of an allergic response, it must weigh at least 1000 Daltons, which is larger than most drugs. Small non-immunogenic molecules, or haptens, may bind to a macromolecular organic carrier to form a conjugate. Such conjugates are chemically active, or if they are activated by biotransformation or photoactivation in the skin [6]. The conjugate can might convert to immunogen and produce a specific humoral, cellular (autoantibody) antibody, or both.

Antibody antigen interaction can take place at the site of drug exposure, causing tissue damage, with an inflammatory reaction as a sign of developing exposure [6–10]. These steps are determined by separate genetic control [11]. A characteristic of this type of drug reactions is that in both animals and humans they occur with a low frequency.

The classification of Gell and Coombs is used frequently [6]. It can be divided into four types of hypersensitivity reactions according to the mechanism of production.

Type I reactions are immediate, anaphylactic, or IgE-mediated reactions. The reaction results from the release of active substances such as: histamine, prostaglandins, platelet-activating factor, leukotrienes, eosinophilic chemotactic factor of IgE-sensitized basophils, and mast cells after contact with the specific antigen. These types of reactions may include systemic anaphylaxis, reactions to insect stings, extrinsic allergic asthma, and some reactions to food.

Type II hypersensitivity reactions represent cytotoxic hypersensitivity, antibody-mediated cytotoxicity, or complement-dependent cytotoxicity [6]. Examples of such reactions are Coombs-positive hemolytic anemia, antibody-mediated thrombocytopenia, leukopenia, pemphigus, pemphigoid, Goodpasture syndrome, leukoclastic vasculitis, and pernicious anemia.

Type III reactions result from the deposition of circulating soluble antigen–antibody complexes in vessels or tissues such as clinical entities in which it is considered that a mechanism of this type may be operating those are drug-induced hepatitis, rheumatoid arthritis, lupus erythematosus, polyarteritis, chronic proliferative membrane glomerulonephritis, and others such as serum disease. The latter, when produced by drugs, as well as forms of kidney disease, are mediated by IgE and are thought to precede type III reactions [6].

Type IV reactions are cell-mediated, with delayed response or tuberculin-type, and are caused by sensitized T lymphocytes after contact with an antigen. Delayed hypersensitivity differs from other forms of sensitivity in that it depends not on antibodies, but on cells. This type of hypersensitivity can be transferred from one sensitive animal to another or from one human to another by administering peripheral blood, its cell extract (transfer factor) but not serum. The clinical entities that are supposed to be related to this type of reaction are contact dermatitis, allograft rejection, several forms of drug sensitivity, and thyroiditis.

A third form of reaction that occurs because of the withdrawal of the drug shall be considered. The most illustrative examples of this type of reaction are the symptoms of withdrawal from narcotics. A reverse reaction is the "rebound" response of exaggerating symptoms that blocked the drug and occurs after abrupt discontinuation of a drug. This is an uncommon response that occurs in the absence or suppression of the drug. Examples of this type of reaction include sympathetic hyperactivity and arterial hypertension following sudden discontinuation of clonidine, or propranolol or adrenal insufficiency following discontinuation of corticosteroids [6].

Another way to classify ADRs is according to their severity, it can classify them as follows [3]:

- Mild; it is one that when it occurs there is no need for therapy or rehabilitation.
- Moderate; it is one that requires a change in pharmacological therapy, although it does not necessarily presuppose the discontinuation of the drug; in this situation, the dose is readjusted, or some other medication may be administered.
- Severe; it is one that requires the discontinuation of the drug and that potentially endangers the life of the subject; it requires specific treatment.
- Lethal; it is one that contributes directly or indirectly to the death of the patient.

According to their prevalence and severity, there are four classes [3, 6]:

1. rare/non-severe, which have little clinical impact...
2. rare/severe, usually identified after the drug is marketed and has administered to many patients...
3. common non-severe and
4. severe common conditions.

Reactions in the latter two categories are part of the pre-FDA approval clinical trials or their equivalent, are listed on the label, and are often part of the risk/benefit ratio in drug choice [12, 13].

ADR can be classified according to the relationship they have with the dose of the medication applied (**Table 1**). Thus, there are adverse reactions that are dose-dependent and others that are not dose-related. The most frequent are the result of an extension of pharmacological effects and can predicted by studies in animals. When an adverse reaction is dose-related, there is almost ample documentation of the effects it produces [12, 13].

Variable	ADR dose-related	ADR no dose-related
Abnormality	Quantitative	Qualitative
Incidence	High	Low
Prediction	Possible	Unpredictable
Presence of liver or kidney disease	Toxicity is increased, depending on the route of elimination of the drug in question	Toxicity is not affected
Prevention of ADR	Dose adjustment	Avoiding the administration of the drug
Treatment	Dose adjustment	Interruption of treatment
Mortality	Usually low	Usually high

Table 1.
Dose-related or not ADR [2, 14].

Another way to classify adverse reactions is according to the organ system affected: blood, skin and annexes, cardiovascular, etc. [3, 6].

One way to make it easier for us to classify adverse reactions is to follow the algorithm in **Table 1**.

4. Factors that predispose to ADRs

How common are adverse reactions? Adverse drug reactions are the most common type of adverse events reported in hospitals [15–23].

There are reports that 19% of all adverse reactions in patients admitted to a hospital were drug-related adverse events [21, 24–28] and are also quite common in outpatients [14] reports that at least 19% of the patients studied in a tertiary medical service had some ADR. Other studies indicate that the incidence of adverse effects varies from 2 to 20%. During a study conducted over an 8-month period, [22] proved that 20% of hospitalized patients developed one or more episodes of ADR. Moreover, in 2% of all patients and 5% of hospitalized patients with complications, iatrogenic disease is considered to contribute to patients' deaths [6].

Adverse reactions are most seen at the extremes of the population, in children and the elderly. There are also reports suggesting that women have a higher number of adverse reactions than men. On the other hand, the existence of a previous adverse reaction to drugs facilitates the presentation of new adverse effects. The simultaneous use of multiple drugs increases the incidence of adverse effects and promotes the occurrence of potentially lethal effects [3, 5, 6, 14, 27].

Prescription drugs are responsible for 90% of the adverse reactions that occur and approximately 7% of ADRs are the result of drug interactions [29].

ADRs are a serious clinical problem both from the point of view of human suffering and from the point of view of costs to the health systems of nations [30]. Bero [31] establishes, based on various studies, that approximately 75% of adverse reactions can be prevented. On the other hand, adequate and early identification of ADR, as well as its reporting or the identification of a therapeutic failure, can easily help to solve the problems, as well as has relevance to the patient, including a reduction in the cost of medical care [21, 32, 33].

According to the Boston Collaborative Drug Surveillance Project [6], the presentation of ADR is considered to lead to hospital admission or strongly influences 3-7% of patients. The same study indicates that in the hospital, the incidence of ADR is 5%; of those, 10% were considered severe. The percentage of deaths caused by a drug was 0.3% (in raw numbers, 1 in 1000 patients).

In addition to the above considerations, it should be taken into account that in most of the studies, especially those carried out in outpatients, it is not known with certainty what other medications the patient was taking; the degree of patient acceptance, as well as the role of excipients, cannot always be obtained and may play an important role in the presentation of ADRs [34].

There are many conditions that can ease the emergence of RAM. One of those factors is age [30, 35, 36]. ADRs are most prevalent at the extremes of life. In the neonate, the liver and kidney enzymes necessary for the metabolism of drugs are not at their best functionality, and therefore, their elimination is less than in adults. In the elderly, degenerative changes in the liver and kidney can hinder the elimination of substances. Alterations in pharmacokinetics found in both neonates and the elderly may facilitate the onset of ADRs.

Another factor is gender. In many studies, it has been established that women have a higher percentage than men of adverse reactions, approximately on the order of 40 to 60% higher [6]. This is thought to be due to many reasons, one of which may be that women may receive more frequent medical care and medications than men. On the other hand, there are periods during a woman's life when there is a physiological alteration that influences the pharmacokinetics of medications, such as menarche, pregnancy, breastfeeding, and menopause [6]. Thus, women may have a higher risk of developing adverse reactions than men.

Patients with an earlier history of ADR may more easily develop adverse reactions [37]. It has been established that 28% of patients with an adverse reaction previously had ADR [6]. A history of allergic disease predisposes to the onset of allergic reactions. It is possible that there is a genetic load that leads to the formation of higher amounts of IgE, increasing the chances of developing anaphylactic-type reactions.

The incidence of ADR increases when multiple drug treatments are being received. This may partly explain the higher number of ADRs found in the elderly. One study estimated that the number of medications taken by a sample of elderly outpatients ranged from 2.8 to 8.3 per day [6]. When multiple medications are taken, there is an increased chance of drug interactions.

Alternatively, the coexistence of diseases may increase the potential for ADR development. A disease involving the kidney and liver leads to the accumulation of the drug in the blood or its toxic metabolites. In a patient with heart disease who is given a potentially cardiotoxic drug, it can more easily lead to the onset of ADRs with more severe effects than would occur in a person with a normal cardiovascular system.

Genetic factors that predominate in some ethnic groups may facilitate predisposition to the occurrence of ADR by polymorphism in drug metabolism and other metabolic variants [6]. For example, there are patients who, due to deficiency of the dehydrogenated glucose-6-phosphate enzyme, have a greater potential to suffer hemolytic episodes when they are administered drugs that alter the redox potential and produce oxidative stress in erythrocytes.

Another important factor to consider is the route of administration, as the bioavailability of substances can be altered; we can cite the poor absorption of drugs administered intramuscularly in a period of shock, the decrease in the absorption of intramuscular phenytoin due to its high pH and precipitation at the site, or the poor response to the hepatitis B vaccine when administered in the gluteal muscle compared to the deltoid muscle [6]. Frequently, due to ignorance of particularities in the absorption of a drug, ADR can be suffered: the administration of drugs through the eye can lead to the systematic absorption of the substance with generalized effects: such is the case of cholinesterase inhibitors.

4.1 Identification of ADR

Information on adverse reactions is generally incomplete when a new drug is introduced to the market. Premarket exposure of a drug is generally in a sample of approximately 1000 to 3000 people (selected, controlled, exclusionary, specific, with no other drug interactions). For this reason, the probability of finding an adverse reaction with a frequency of occurrence less than 1:1000 is remote. In addition, patient inclusion criteria associated with controlled clinical trials generally do not allow for a good estimate of the frequency of some ADRs in subgroups of patients with accompanying complications or diseases or receiving multiple medications.

For the above reasons, the full range of ADRs may not be adequately established until the following conditions are met [4, 23]: (which characterize the general population using the drug in question).

1. administration to patients with a diversity of diseases or physiological or pathological conditions.

2. administration to hundreds or thousands of patients, especially for the identification of ADRs with an incidence of less than 1:10000 and

3. Administration for extended periods of time.

It should also be noted that ADR can become evident long after the administration of the drug has ceased, as is the case with cancer developed in the daughters of mothers who ingested diethylstilbestrol during pregnancy.

For the above reasons, the full range of ADRs may not be established until the drug has been marketed and only with the time.

The previous paragraphs lead us to think that the correct identification of an ADR can help not only the knowledge of the drug [38], but, more importantly, the alleviation of patients' suffering [4, 23].

There is no method that ensures the correct identification of a RAM. It is not always easy to prove the cause-and-effect relationship between the administration of a drug and the onset of ADR. However, there are some recommendations that can guide us in this regard. [13, 39] suggest some criteria that may help us find an adverse event:

1. Ensure that there is a temporal sequence between the administration of the drug and the onset of the adverse event

2. The adverse event must be related to the pharmacological or adverse effects of the drug. It should be ensured that the non-drug therapy or the patient's disease does not produce such ADR.

Check what happens if the patient, accidentally or intentionally, takes the drug again.

5. Causality

The establishment of causality is one of the most critical problems faced by a researcher when trying to evaluate the role of a drug in the development of ADR. This is due to several situations.

First, the body has a limited range of response to aggression. Therefore, ADR may be clinically like the clinical expression of other pathologies not caused by drugs. Therefore, this similarity between ADR and the symptomatology of a disease makes it difficult to differentiate between a causal association and a pathology.

In clinical trials in large numbers of patients, a large sample size may be sufficient for causality to be proven with the help of statistics. However, this occurs in the fewest of cases. When faced with a single event, the "clinical judgment" is responsible for determining the existing association [3].

Clinical judgment is usually based on the physician's experience as well as knowledge; but both factors can be highly variable between doctors and even within the same doctor at different stages of their life. We often find disagreements regarding the interpretation of causality among different experts in the field [39, 40].

Due to this variation in the interpretation of the data, some methods have been established that help decision-making in a structured and standardized way.

In 1981, Naranjo et al. [41, 42], published a method consisting of assigning a series of scores based on the answer to some questions. The sum of the scores leads to an overall punctuation that determines the relationship between the drug and ADRs, differentiating their relationship between certain or definitive, or probable, or possible or doubtful [3].

The characterization of each of the above categories could be established as follows [41, 42].

Definitive: A reaction that:

1. Occur in a reasonable time sequence after administration of the drug or in which levels of the drug have been established in body fluids or tissues.

2. follows a known response pattern for the drug.

3. is confirmed by improvement after discontinuation of the drug or worsening when readministering the drug, and

4. which cannot be explained by the known characteristics of the patient's disease.

Probable: A reaction that:

1. It has a reasonable time sequence after administration of the drug.

2. follows a known response pattern.

3. is confirmed by discontinuation of the drug, but not by reinstatement of treatment, and

4. which cannot be explained by the characteristics of the patient's disease.

Possible:

1. It has a reasonable time sequence after administration of the drug.

2. may or may not follow a known response pattern, but

3. which can be explained by the characteristics of the patient's disease.

However, many physicians disagree with the previous method; this is why other techniques have been developed, such as the Bayesian Adverse Reaction Diagnostic Instrument (BARDI), which considers the evaluation of the causality of an ADR to be a special case of conditional probability. The application of this method has been simplified through the development of analysis by computational methods.

Adverse drug reactions (ADRs) are responsible around for 10% of outpatient appointments [43, 44] and 3.5–10% of hospital admissions [43, 44] and are the fifth leading cause of death in hospitalized patients, in addition to prolonging stays and presenting a high economic impact [45]. The spontaneous reporting of suspected ADRs by health professionals allows continuous determination of the benefit–risk ratio of a given drug and is one of the best methods to generate signals on unexpected events and rare ADRs [15].

5.1 Adverse drug reactions in Mexico

In 1999, Mexico joined the WHO Program for International Drug Monitoring Center coordinated by the WHO and, ever since, the National Pharmacovigilance Center (CNF–Centro Nacional de Farmacovigilancia) is responsible for coordinating pharmacovigilance activities in the country, supported by an organization in which the Institutional Pharmacovigilance Centers, the State Pharmacovigilance Centers, and the Pharmaceutical Industry participate. Mexico has been a member of the Program for International Drug Monitoring coordinated by World Health Organization since 1999 [46].

The National program is specifically regulated by the Mexican Official Norm, NOM-220-SSA1-2012, "Pharmacovigilance Installation and Operation", which points out as mandatory the notification of adverse drug reactions and the NOM-240-SSA1-2012, intended for medical devices, which was launched in October 2012, both involving institutions of public and private sectors of the National Health System, as well as healthcare professionals, the owner of marketing registry or their legal representative, establishments dedicated to the sale and supply of medicinal products, and clinical research units.

'The Pharmacovigilance Guide for Notification of Suspected Adverse Drug Reactions' [47] define pharmacovigilance as activities related to the detection, evaluation, understanding and prevention of adverse events, suspected adverse reactions, adverse reactions, events allegedly attributable to vaccination or immunization, or any other safety problem related to the use of medicines and vaccines [47].

The NOM-220-SSA1-2012 was updated in 2016 and recently in 2024. According to Mexican NOM-220, the aims are detection, identification, quantification, evaluation, and prevention of the possible risks derived from the use of medicines in humans. To evaluate the safety of the medicines or vaccines that are marketed in the country and protect the health of the Mexican population, it is necessary to subject them to continuous monitoring if they are available.

The main report of pharmacovigilance is the spontaneous report of adverse drug reactions by the physicians and the health professionals [5, 48–50]. In Mexico, any spontaneous report can be sent directly to the health authority or through entities that collect and register the reports, known as state-centers, or pharmacovigilance institutional centers, the pharmaceutical industry, and clinical research units, who, as well as health professionals and medications users, provide information to the health authority [48, 51]. One of the major drawbacks of spontaneous reporting of suspected ADRs is underreporting [6, 44, 45, 52–54]. Indeed, it is estimated that only 6%of all ADRs are reported [55]. Underreporting delays the triggering of signals and, by extension, the decisions to maintain an appropriate drug benefit-to-harm balance. Any one of a series of factors may account for underreporting, including knowledge, attitudes, lack of time, and respondent's motivation [49]. While e-Reporting Industry is free to acquire, MedDRA and WHODrug licenses generate an annual update and additional cost. This makes it difficult to use this tool to facilitate spontaneous reporting by physicians and other health professionals. Therefore, it continues to be sent directly to the health authority or entities that collect the reports, making inadequate and timely approval of the notification.

For a population of 126 million inhabitants (INEGI, 2020), Mexico should generate at least 25,200 useful notifications each year. The fact is that this goal had only recent achieved due to the bad quality of the reports generated in the past and to the lack of feedback to the reporters.

As observed in 2009 [46], there were 26,640 notifications reported, but only 11,284 became useful reports. The origin of the reports involved the pharmaceutical industry (58%), state centers (11%), institutional centers (3%), healthcare professionals directly to health authority (0.5%), medication consumers (0.5%), and adverse events coming from clinical research (27%) (not necessarily associated with drugs). Unfortunately, the quality of information issued by the pharmaceutical industry was inappropriate in 77% of the cases.

In a high percentage of the notifications, the quality of the information is not good, and the lack of feedback has not allowed improvement. Despite the tasks performed having evolved, they still do not have an impact on public health. In general, information in the study samples of the suspected ADR reports sent to the CNFV during 2007 and 2010 was incomplete and did not fulfill the requirements established by the NOM guidelines [51]. Among the CEFV, pharmaceutical industry, and CIFV, the suspected ADR reports were mainly provided by pharmaceutical industries. According to the information completeness classification categories used, most of the suspected ADR reports from the pharmaceutical industry were classified as grade 0 (provided information was insufficient to generate risk signals). The seriousness of most of the suspected ADR reports was classified as non-serious; however, about 2% were found to be fatal [51]. It seems necessary to improve the pharmacovigilance system in Mexico and to promote submission of high completeness of suspected ADR reports that fully fulfill the Mexican NOM specifications. These measures are necessary to generate risk signals and prevent ADRs [48, 56]. However, since 2023, the health authorities in Mexico are working together with UMC, to promote adequate and timely approval notifications.

In general, the physician underestimates adverse reactions to medications, although there is a group of health professionals who are at the other extreme. Any of these attitudes can be as dangerous to the patient as the adverse reactions themselves [3, 6, 7, 24, 52, 57–61]; underreporting is a major limitation of spontaneous notification systems, and as mentioned before, it is estimated that only 6–10% of all ADRs are reported [52]. On the one hand, this high underreporting rate prevents ADRs from being quantified to calculate their impact in terms of incidence and risk [14], and on the other hand, it delays the activation of warning signals, with the consequent repercussions on public health [49, 52, 55, 62].

Low ADR reporting is still associated with a series of attitudes (ignorance, lack of confidence, or complacency) and excuses that are potentially modifiable through training or by facilitating the notification process [57]. This suggests that over the last decade there have been low significant advances in the training of health professionals on ADR reporting and that it is necessary for health systems and (academy/training levels, or courses) centers to deepen the training of health professionals about drug safety [15, 63]. This would provide a greater capacity to activate early warnings to the pharmacovigilance systems and thus allow the health authorities to react more quickly to ensure that the least possible number of patients are affected. Also, the universities must reinforce in the health professionals the education in pharmacovigilance. Recent observations are in concordance, not only in Mexico but around the world [56, 64, 65].

The health professional need to improve (a) access to an efficient reporting mechanism and (b) knowledge of what and how to report an ADR to engage and promote the reporting of ADRs.

Physicians' underreporting of adverse drug reactions (ADRs) can be attributed to several factors: Fear of Punitive or Legal Ramifications:

Physicians may hesitate to report ADRs due to concerns about potential legal consequences or punitive actions, even when assured of anonymity.

Lack of Instruction During Training: Insufficient training on ADR reporting processes can hinder physicians from recognizing and reporting adverse events effectively.

Excessive Paperwork and Time Constraints: The administrative burden associated with reporting ADRs, including paperwork and time requirements, can discourage physicians from actively participating in the reporting process.

Incentive Gap: The absence of incentives or rewards for reporting ADRs may contribute to underreporting. Physicians may prioritize other clinical tasks over reporting ADRs due to the lack of tangible benefits.

Addressing these barriers and promoting a positive reporting culture can help improve ADR reporting among healthcare professionals [57]. If you suspect an adverse reaction to a drug or medical device, it is essential to fulfill your ethical responsibility by reporting it.

In Mexico, pharmacovigilance activities became compulsory in 2012 after publication of the Official Mexican Standard NOM-220-SSA1-2012 and its updates in 2016 and 2024; "Establishment and Operation of Pharmacovigilance", [47] which requires that all hospitals establish a Pharmacovigilance Unit (PVU), led by the Head of Pharmacovigilance (HP), who must be a health professional, with the commission of providing notifications of ADRs to the State Center for Pharmacovigilance (SCPV), which reports to the Pharmacovigilance National Center [63]. Health professionals reported suspected ADR by using "The Suspect Adverse Drug Reaction to Medicines Notice Form" published on the webpage of the Federal Commission for the Protection Against Sanitary Risks. The HP reviewed the forms to assess whether they fulfilled the criteria for valid notification, according to "The Pharmacovigilance Guide for Notification of Suspected Adverse Drug Reactions" [47]. If the information was incomplete, the HP communicated with the reporting health professional to complete the report. If the reporter did not complete the information, the PVU did not accept the notification. Reports were categorized as incomplete if they lacked information such as medication brand, production batch, or expiration date. As established by the National Health System of Mexico, notifications shall be submitted in no more than 30 calendar days after their identification, for severe drug reactions (drug reactions that interfere with the habitual activities of the patient, require suspension of the medication and the administration of rescue medications), or in no more than 90 calendar days after their identification, for not severe drug reactions. Reporting excludes intentional or accidental poisoning, drugs abuse, and adverse events due to errors in drug administration or patient non-compliance of pharmacotherapy. Unfortunately, health budget cuts and the implementation of effective government programs represent a challenge for Mexico. These restrictions affect all healthcare levels in Mexico.

Notifications that fulfilled all the requirements were sent through an informatics platform. Overlooking an ADR could result in the provision of inappropriate treatment for such reactions. The global prevalence of underreporting of ADEs is a major cause for concern. Such underreporting can lead to delays in identifying safety issues associated with drugs and cause harm to patients. Additionally, it can prevent identification of flaws in the medication delivery process, posing further drug safety risks. It is worth noting that even in countries with advanced healthcare systems, the underreporting of ADEs persists, indicating that the issue is not solely related to inadequate infrastructure or resources. Thus, maintaining vigilance in identifying and diagnosing ADRs is critical. Such vigilance is achieved through the collaborative efforts of a multidisciplinary healthcare team and the expedite communication of all parties involved in the process of pharmacovigilance.

Author details

Miguel Luján Estrada[1*], Aivle Libertad Hernández Caamaño[2] and Karla Roman Flores[1]

1 Unidad de Farmacovigilancia, Grupo Bruluart, Geranios, Col. San Francisco Chilpan, C.P., Tultitlan, Estado de México, México

2 Pharmet, S.A de C.V. Avenida de las Granjas, Col. Santa Bárbara, Azcapotzalco, Ciudad de México, México

*Address all correspondence to: miglujan@hotmail.com

IntechOpen

© 2024 The Author(s). Licensee IntechOpen. This chapter is distributed under the terms of the Creative Commons Attribution License (http://creativecommons.org/licenses/by/4.0), which permits unrestricted use, distribution, and reproduction in any medium, provided the original work is properly cited.

References

[1] Seifert R. Drugs Easily Explained. Switzerland AG: Springer Nature; 2022. pp. 1-267. DOI: 10.1007/978-3-031-12188-3

[2] Spilker B, Cuatrecasas P. Inside the Drug Industry. Publication/Creation Barcelona: Prous Science Publishers; 1990. 109 p

[3] Portoles A, Vargas E. Reacciones adversas a medicamentos. In: Velásquez. Farmacología. 16th ed. N.Y. USA: Interamericana McGraw-Hill; 1993. pp. 92-107

[4] World Health Organization. The importance of pharmacovigilance: Safety monitoring of medical products [online]. Available from: http://www.ops.org.bo/textocompleto/ime18633.pdf [Accessed: May 12, 2023]

[5] Rabbur RSM, Emmerton L. An introduction to adverse drug reaction reporting systems in different countries. International Journal of Pharmacy Practice. 2005;**13**:91-10

[6] Glazener F. Adverse drug reactions. In: Melmon and Morreli's Clinical Pharmacology. Basis Principles in Therapeutics. 3th ed. McGraw-Hill, Inc. USA; 1992. pp. 977-1011

[7] Pohl LR et al. The immunological and metabolic basis of drug hypersensitivities. Annual Review of Pharmacology and Toxicology. 1988;**28**:367-387

[8] Park BK et al. Idiosyncratic drug reactions: A mechanistic evaluation of risk factors. British Journal of Clinical Pharmacology. 1992;**34**:377-395

[9] Parker CW. Drug allergy. The New England Journal of Medicine. 1975;**292**:957-960

[10] Pasricha JS. Drugs causing fixed eruptions. The British Journal of Dermatology. 1979;**100**:183-185

[11] Benacerraf B. Role of MHC gene products in immune regulation. Science. 1981;**212**:1229-1238

[12] Karch FE, Lasagna L. Adverse drug reactions a critical review. JAMA. 1975;**234**:1236-1241

[13] Karch FE, Lasagna L. Toward the operational identification of adverse drug reactions. Clinical Pharmacology and Therapeutics. 1977;**21**:247-254

[14] Rabelo-Melo JR, Duarte EC, de Araujo FK, et al. Under-reporting of adverse drug reactions among healthcare professionals in Brazil: An estimate based on National pharmacovigilance survey. Journal of Young Pharmacists. 2020;**12**(4):360-365

[15] Bandekar MS, Anwikar SR, Kshirsagar NA. Quality check of spontaneous adverse drug reaction reporting forms of different countries. Pharmacoepidemiology and Drug Safety. 2010;**19**:1181-1185

[16] Davies EC, Green CF, Mottram DR, Pirmohamed M. Adverse drug reactions in hospitals: A narrative review. Current Drug Safety. 2007;**2**:79-87

[17] Emerson A, Martin MR, Tomlin M, et al. Prospective cohort study of adverse events monitored by hospital pharmacists. Pharmacoepidemiology and Drug Safety. 2001;**10**:95-103

[18] Hartwig SC et al. Preventability and severity assessment in reporting adverse drug reactions. American Journal of Hospital Pharmacy. 1992;**49**:2229-2232

[19] Laporte JR, Carne´ X. Epidemiological basic methodology in pharmacovigilance. In: Laporte JR, Tognoni G, editors. Drug Epidemiology Principles. 2nd ed. Barcelona: Masson-Salvat; 1993. pp. 111-127

[20] Lazarou J et al. Incidence of adverse drug reactions in hospitalized patients a meta-analysis of prospective studies. JAMA. 1998;**279**:1200

[21] Leape LL et al. The nature of adverse events in hospitalized patients: Results of the Harvard medical practice study II. The New England Journal of Medicine. 1991;**324**:377-384

[22] Schimmel EM. The hazards of hospitalization. Annals of Internal Medicine. 1964;**60**:100-110

[23] WHO. Policy perspectives on medicines — Pharmacovigilance: Ensuring the safe use of medicines. 2004. pp. 1-6

[24] Brennan TA. Incidence of adverse events and negligence in hospitalized patients: Results of the Harvard medical practice study. The New England Journal of Medicine. 1991;**324**:370-376

[25] Kennedy DL et al. Monitoring of adverse drug events in hospitals. JAMA. 1991;**266**:28-78

[26] Kessler DA. Introducing MEDWatch: A new approach to reporting medication and device adverse effects and product problems. JAMA. 1993;**269**:2765-2768

[27] Sukanta Sen SK, Rahaman R, Chatterjee D, et al. Knowledge, attitudes and practice of adverse drug reaction monitoring among physicians in India. International Journal of Basic & Clinical Pharmacology. 2017;**6**:1497-1506. DOI: 10.18203/2319-2003.ijbcp20172249

[28] Waller PC. Measuring the frequency of adverse drug reactions. British Journal of Clinical Pharmacology. 1992;**33**:249-252

[29] Edlavitch SA. Adverse drug event reporting: Improving the low US reporting rates, editorial. Archives of Internal Medicine. 1988;**148**:1499-1503

[30] Bero LA et al. Characterization of geriatric drug-related hospital readmissions. Medical Care. 1991;**29**:989-1003

[31] Dukes MNG. Economic costs of adverse drug reactions. Pharmacoeconomics. 1992;**1**:153-154

[32] Gonzalez-Gonzalez C, Lopez-Gonzalez E, Herdeiro MT, Figueiras A. Strategies to improve adverse drug reaction reporting: A critical and systematic review. Drug Safety. 2013;**36**:317-328

[33] Mirjam K, Rommers MK, Teepe-Twiss IM, et al. Preventing adverse drug events in hospital practice: An overview. Pharmacoepidemiology and Drug Safety. 2007;**10**:1-7

[34] Lockey SD. Reactions to hidden agents in foods, beverages, and drugs. Annals of Allergy. 1971;**29**:461-466

[35] Chrischilles EA et al. Self-reported adverse drug reactions and related resource use: A study of community-dwelling persons 65 years of age and older. Annals of Internal Medicine. 1992;**117**:634-640

[36] Gurwitz JH, Avorn J. The ambiguous relation between aging and adverse drug reactions. Annals of Internal Medicine. 1991;**114**:956-966

[37] Saxon A, Beall GN, Rohr AS, Adelman DC. Immediate hypersensitivity

reactions to beta-lactam antibiotics and penicillin in penicillin-allergic subjects. The Journal of Infectious Diseases. 1984;**149**:16-22

[38] Saladrigas MV. El sistema de clasificacion ATC de sustancias farmacéuticas para uso humano. Panacea [Online]. 2004;**5**:58-60

[39] Karch FE, Smith CL, Kerzner B, Mazzullo JM, Weintrub M, Lasagna L. Adverse drug reaction-a matter of opinion. Clinical Pharmacology and Therapeutics. 1976;**19**:489-492

[40] Koch-Weser J, Sellers EM, Zacest R. The ambiguity of adverse drug reactions. European Journal of Clinical Pharmacology. 1977;**11**:75-78

[41] Naranjo CA, Busto U. Adverse drug reactions. In: Kalant/Roschlau. Principles of Medical Pharmacology. 5th ed. Toronto, Can: B.C. Decker Ing; 1989. pp. 658-665

[42] Naranjo CA, Busto U, Sellers EM, et al. A method for estimating probability of adverse drug reactions. Clinical Pharmacology and Therapeutics. 1981;**30**:239-245

[43] Davies EC, Green CF, Taylor S, Williamson PR, Mottram DR, Pirmohamed M. Adverse drug reactions in hospital In-patients: A prospective analysis of 3695 patient-episodes. PLoS One. 2009;**4**(2):e4439. DOI: 10.1371/journal.pone.0004439

[44] Formica D, Sultana J, Cutroneo PM, Lucchesi S, Angelica R, et al. The economic burden of preventable adverse drug reactions: A systematic review of observational studies. Expert Opinion on Drug Safety. 2018;**17**:681-695. DOI: 10.1080/14740338.2018.1491547

[45] Bouvy JC, De Bruin ML, Koopmanschap MA. Epidemiology of adverse drug reactions in Europe: A review of recent observational studies. Drug Safety. 2015;**38**:437-453

[46] Rosete A, Benítez-Vázquez R. Spontaneous reporting in Mexico. In: Andrews EB, Moore N, editors. Mann's Pharmacovigilance. 3rd ed. John Wiley & Sons, Ltd; 2014. Available from: www.wiley.com\go\mann\pharmacovigilance

[47] NOM-220-SA1-2012, and NOM-220-SA1-2016, Norma Oficial Mexicana. Instalacion y Operación de la Farmacovigilancia [Online] 2012. Available from: www.dof.gob.mx/nota_detalle.php?codigo=5284236&fecha=07/01/2013 [Accessed: December 10, 2023]

[48] Rayon Ramirez G, Alvarado López S, Camacho Sandoval R, Loera MJ, et al. Strengthening the pharmacovigilance system in Mexico: Implementation of VigiFlow and VigiLyze, as ICSR and signal detection management systems. Pharmaceutical Medicine. 2023;**37**:425-437

[49] Lopez-Gonzalez E, Herdeiro MT, Figueiras A. Determinants of under-reporting of adverse drug reactions: A systematic review. Drug Safety. 2009;**32**:19-31

[50] Salvador MR, Monteiro C, Pereira L, Duarte AP. Quality of spontaneous reports of adverse drug reactions sent to a regional pharmacovigilance unit. International Journal of Environmental Research and Public Health. 2022;**19**(7):3754. DOI: 10.3390/ijerph19073754

[51] Sánchez-Sánchez B, Altagracia-Martínez M, Kravzov-Jinich J, et al. Evaluation of completeness of suspected adverse drug reaction reports submitted to the Mexican national pharmacovigilance centre.

A cross-sectional period-prevalence study. Drug Safety. 2012;**35**(10):837-844

[52] Al Meslamani AZ. Underreporting of adverse drug events: A look into the extent, causes, and potential solutions. Expert Opinion on Drug Safety. 2023;**22**(5):351-354

[53] Faich GA et al. National adverse drug reaction surveillance: 1985. JAMA. 1986;**257**:2068-2070

[54] Garcia Abeijon P, Costa C, Taracido M, Herdeiro MT, et al. Factors associated with underreporting of adverse drug reactions by health care professionals: A systematic review update. Drug Safety. 2023;**46**:625-636

[55] Hazell L, Shakir SAW. Under-reporting of adverse drug reactions. A systematic review. Drug Safety. 2006;**29**(5):385-396

[56] Reumerman M, Tichellar J, Piersma B, et al. Urgent need to modernize pharmacovigilance education in healthcare curricula: Review of the literature. European Journal of Clinical Pharmacology. 2018;**74**:1235-1248

[57] Al-Worafi YM. Chapter 5. Adverse drug reactions. In: Drug Safety in Developing Countries. Achievements and Challenges. Elsevier Inc; 2020. pp. 39-57. DOI: 10.1016/B978-0-12-819837-7.00005-4

[58] Ekman E, Bäckström M. Attitudes among hospital physicians to the reporting of adverse drug reactions in Sweden. European Journal of Clinical Pharmacology. 2008;**65**(1):43-46

[59] Strom BL, Tugwell P. Pharmacoepidemiology: Current status, prospects, and problems. Annals of Internal Medicine. 1990;**113**:179-181

[60] Valdez-Ramirez AL et al. Implementation of the pharmacovigilance unit in a Mexican hospital. Journal of Pharmacy Practice and Research. 2018;**48**:583-584

[61] Valdez-Ramırez LA, Serrano-Medina A, Cornejo-Bravo JM. Adverse drug reactions' reporting in a Mexican hospital. International Journal of Pharmacy Practice. 2020;**28**(6):660-662. DOI: 10.1111/ijpp.12639

[62] Moride Y, Requejo HF, AA and Begaud B. Under-reporting of adverse drug reactions in general practice. British Journal of Clinical Pharmacology. 1997;**43**:177-181

[63] Ashish K, Kuperman GJ, Rittemberg E, et al. Identifying hospital admissions due to adverse drug events using a computer-based monitor. Pharmacoepidemiology and Drug Safety. 2001;**10**:113-119

[64] Herrera CR. Undergraduate and postgraduate pharmacovigilance education: A proposal for appropriate curriculum content. British Journal of Clinical Pharmacology. 2020;**86**:779-790

[65] Herrera CJ, Núñez LME. Pharmacovigilance. In: Herrera CJ, editor. Handbook of Clinical Pharmacy and Pharmaceutical Care. 1st ed. Madrid: Elsevier; 2003. pp. 283-296